the total
kettlebell workout

TRADE SECRETS OF A PERSONAL TRAINER

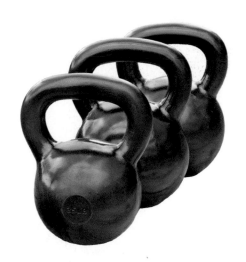

Published by Bloomsbury Publishing Plc
50 Bedford Square
London WC1B 3DP
www.bloomsbury.com

First edition 2013

ISBN (print): 978 1 4088 3257 8
ISBN (epub): 978 1 4081 9373 0
ISBN (epdf): 978 1 4081 9374 7

Acknowledgements
Cover photograph © Esc Creative LLP www.esccreative.com
Inside photographs © Esc Creative LLP for exercise photos;
all filler images © Shutterstock
Illustrations by David Gardner
Commissioning Editor: Charlotte Croft
Editor: Sarah Cole
Cover and textual designer: James Watson

This book is produced using paper that is made from wood grown in managed, sustainable forests. It is natural, renewable and recyclable. The logging and manufacturing processes conform to the environmental regulations of the country of origin.

Typeset in 10.25pt on 13.5pt URWGroteskLig by Margaret Brain, Wisbech

Printed and bound in India by Replika Press Pvt Ltd

10 9 8 7 6 5 4 3 2 1

the total
kettlebell workout

TRADE SECRETS OF A PERSONAL TRAINER

STEVE BARRETT

BLOOMSBURY

LONDON · NEW DELHI · NEW YORK · SYDNEY

disclaimer and advisory

Before attempting any form of exercise, especially that which involves lifting weights, always ensure you have a safe working environment. Ensure that the floor surface you are on is non-slip and do not stand on any rugs or mats that could move when you exercise. Also, clear your exercise space of items that could cause you harm if you collided with them; this includes furniture, pets and children. Pay particular attention to the amount of clearance you have above your head and remember that for some of the exercise moves you will be raising your hands and the weights above head height, so keep away from doorways and light fittings.

The information, workouts, health related information and activities described in this publication are practiced and developed by the author and should be used as an adjunct to your understanding of health and fitness and, in particular, strength training. While physical exercise is widely acknowledged as being beneficial to a participant's health and well-being, the activities and methods outlined in this book may not be appropriate for everyone. It is fitness industry procedure to recommend all individuals, especially those suffering from disease or illness, to consult their doctor for advice on their suitability to follow specific types of activity. This advice also applies to any person who has experienced soft tissue or skeletal injuries in the past, those who have recently received any type of medical treatment or are taking medication and women who are, or think they may be, pregnant.

The author has personally researched and tried all of the exercises, methods and advice given in this book on himself and with many training clients. However, this does not mean these activities are universally appropriate and neither he nor the publishers are, therefore, liable or responsible for any injury, distress or harm that you consider may have resulted from following the information contained in this publication.

contents

1 the basics of exercising with kettlebells

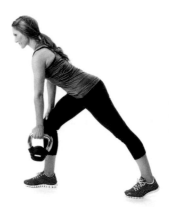

the S.A.F.E. trainer system
(Simple, Achievable, Functional Exercise)

We need to exercise our bodies in a way that is achievable, effective and, most of all, sustainable so that the method becomes part of our lifestyle, rather than an inconvenience.

In a perfect world everyone would be able to lift their own bodyweight above their head, have ideal body-fat levels and be able to run a four-minute mile. Any one of these goals is achievable if you are highly motivated and have very few other commitments in your life, but the reality is that most people are so far off this state of perfection that the biggest challenge is either starting an exercise programme, or staying committed and engaged with a method of training for long enough to see any kind of improvement.

Exercise is in many ways a perfect product, because it has very few negative side effects, it is cheap to do and highly versatile. But so many high profile, quick-fix programmes and products make exercise sound easy, as though it is a magic wand that once waved will bring near instant results. And with the fitness industry constantly driven by innovation in products and methods, the diverse and sometimes bewildering amount of advice available makes it all too easy to be overwhelmed. The truth is that many training programmes and methods will theoretically work, but the level of commitment needed is so high that when you add in work and family responsibilities, stress and other demands upon time, most of us simply cannot stick to a plan.

I also find that those programmes which seem too good to be true usually have a series of components that are not explicit in the headline, but are required to achieve the spectacular results they boast about. So you sign up to a workout programme claiming: 'Instant fat loss – ultra 60 second workout!' only to find that to achieve the promised weight loss you have to go on an impossible 500-calories-a-day diet. These methods also assume that everybody is fairly perfect already; by this I mean they don't have any injuries, they are strong, mobile and flexible and have a cardiovascular system that will soak up anaerobic training from day one. If these people are out there, I don't see them walking up and down the average high street. There is a real need to approach fitness in a more down to earth, less sensationalist way. We need to exercise our bodies in a

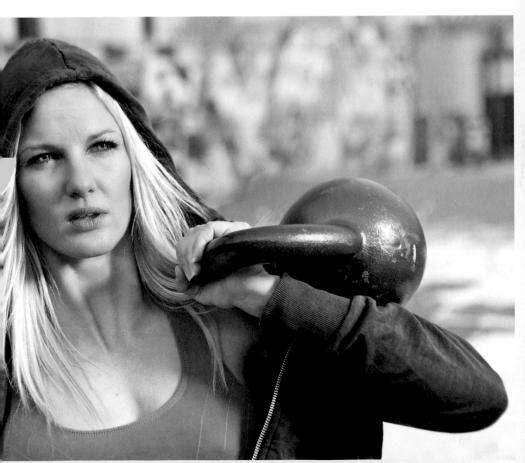

way that is achievable, effective and, most of all, sustainable so that the method becomes part of our lifestyle, rather than an inconvenience.

My S.A.F.E. trainer system (Simple, Achievable, Functional Exercise) is all of these things. It is based on 20 years of personal training experience, including many thousands of hours of coaching, lifting, running, jumping and stretching with people from all walks of life, from the average man or woman to elite athletes. My system respects the natural way that the body adapts to activity and creates a perfect physiological learning curve.

All S.A.F.E. trainer system moves develop stability, strength or power. If you're not familiar with these essential components of human performance, I am sure that you will recognise the saying: 'You have to walk before you can run'. This is the epitome of my approach, because when a client says they want to run or jump, the first thing I have to establish as a personal trainer is that they are at least already at the walking stage. I consider stability to be the walking phase of human movement, as it teaches you the correct muscle recruitment patterns; strength the running phase, as it trains the body to do these moves against a greater force (resistance); and power the jumping phase, since it teaches you to add speed and dynamics to the movement.

So, where do kettlebells fit in? Well, at this stage of most books you will be under no illusion that the author is fanatical about this form of training and that he or she believes that their methods are the solution to everybody's health and fitness problems. In many cases I would agree because any kind of exercise is better than no exercise, however, simply grabbing a kettlebell and swinging it around like you have seen the guys do at the gym is a fast track route to an injury. Therefore, with this product more than any other I find myself asking if a client is really ready. In my opinion, kettlebells are not suitable for 'absolute' beginners to exercise. I know the purist will wave testimonials featuring success stories, but for every one of those there will be a forgotten individual who did too much too soon and sustained an injury to their back or shoulder. Even those of us who do move our bodies frequently need to consider some pre-conditioning before grabbing a kettlebell because a good level of cardiovascular fitness and strength will not automatically predispose you to be ready for the advanced challenges that kettlebells can inflict upon the body.

Why not? Inertia! Depending upon the length of your limbs, when a kettlebell is swung through an arc the mass is multiplied by between three and four times the weight of the kettlebell so the 16kg weight that you grabbed for your first session feels more like 64kg at the top of the movement! Is this a problem? Well it shouldn't be and probably won't be for most experienced strength athletes (like the ones you normally see in kettlebell books) unlike the people who are 'work in progress' that personal trainers normally deal with. Kettlebells have gone from being a niche product used by hardcore 'strong man' athletes to being a mainstream fitness product that can be purchased in supermarkets alongside much 'softer' fitness products like mats, skipping ropes and ridiculously small dumbbells. And that is where the problems begin – despite being the epitome of simplicity, a kettlebell has more potential to hurt you than any other fitness product, yet I still see personal trainers getting de-conditioned, immobile clients to swing the weights around in the gym with techniques that leave a lot to be desired.

Interestingly, kettlebells have become accepted as a part of the mainstream fitness industry in a way that doesn't compare to any other method of exercise – in my 20 plus years as part of the fitness industry whenever a new type of exercise is launched there is always a scientific study that can be quoted or scored to validate the methods used. However, with kettlebells it is very hard to find any conclusive independent research (by which I mean research not carried out by training companies or equipment manufacturers) that gives clear, subjective advice as to how, when and what an individual should do with a kettlebell. There are two main reasons for this. Firstly, there is no commercial motivation to conduct research into training methods which are already commercially available. Secondly, any studies that were conducted would be very subjective because with kettlebell movements the individual user gets a unique experience based on their anatomical characteristics (height and length of limbs). So, unless the study included hundreds or thousands of individuals through a wide spectrum of body shapes, the information would be extremely subjective – basically, a 140cm tall person swinging a 16kg weight will get a completely different sensation and set of forces than a 165cm tall person swinging the same 16kg weight.

Many of the exercises performed with kettlebells were originally conceived to strengthen individuals who had reached a point in their training where the only challenge was to keep adding more and more weight to barbells, and while there is nothing wrong with that ultimately they would become a different kind of athlete. This book focuses on all the positive reasons for using kettlebells and aims to help you enhance the results you get from the time you spend doing strength and conditioning training but I also aim to add some structure to the use of kettlebells which extends beyond the usual approach to using them which seems to be a 'one size fits all' approach.

When you get to the portfolio of exercises (see page 41) demonstrating the actual exercises (or 'moves' as I like to call them) you will find that, rather than just being a list of exercises with kettlebells, I have focused on the moves that really work and you may be surprised by the order in which I present them. Most books seem to ignore the fact that the first time you swing a kettlebell is often the first time that ligaments and tendons have experienced such forces, so I don't start with the classic swing moves as my intention is to break you in more gently and to give the body an opportunity to 'pre'-condition itself before being exposed to the exercises which play with the effects of inertia. My moves can be done with either a single weight or preferably a selection of kettlebells ranging from 8kg up to 32kg. There are hundreds of moves that can be done with a kettlebell, but many of them are very similar to each other, often ineffective or sometimes potentially dangerous. This book is all about combining skills and methods to create safe and effective fitness ideas to help you get the most out of the time you invest in exercise.

You'll find that the majority of the exercises progress through three stages; I don't like to refer to these as easy, medium and advanced because in reality some of the changes are very subtle while on others you would really notice if you were to try all three versions back to back. Instead, the following three levels closely mirror the systematic approach athletes use in the weight training room and on the training field:

1 each move can be progressed or regressed by changing body position;
2 resistance is applied to the move;
3 the speed at which the move is performed is increased;
– or in fact a combination of all three.

Remember, if you're moving, you're improving.

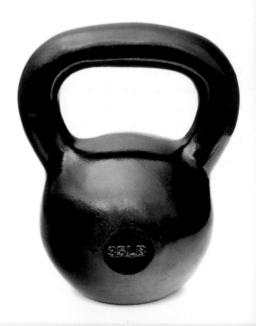

how to use this book

To help you make sense of each kettlebell activity and how it relates to my S.A.F.E. training system, each move is classified by its respective outcome, whether that is an increase in stability, strength or power, rather than the more subjective easy, medium and hard.

Training with kettlebells is an efficient use of your time. Clearly, the amount of time you spend active will dictate the outcomes, however, of all the pieces of fitness equipment available, kettlebells have the ability to be unintentionally 'traumatic' to the muscle, ligaments and tendons. So there is a fine balance between doing too much too soon and not giving the body long enough to recover between sessions. Therefore, greater results are likely if you also aim for quality rather than sheer quantity.

When I started to think about writing this book, the first thing I had to come to terms with is that there are many other books available that set out to teach you how to use kettlebells, with many of them written by very good trainers who have a fanatical approach to their use. Likewise, in my everyday life as a personal trainer I know that my clients have access to information not only from myself, but from a wide range of sources such as the web, books and no doubt other personal trainers they come across in the gym, therefore it may turn out that my approach differs from others and in particular that I have a more cautious approach to using kettlebells than them. That's fine with me as I would rather have a client who needed to work for a few more weeks or months to reach their goals rather than one who becomes injured because they were given ambitious advice.

As I have worked with many of my clients now for over a decade, clearly they find my approach productive and a worthwhile investment. With this in mind, my aim is to condense 25 years' experience of training my own body and, more importantly, 20 years' experience as a personal trainer and many thousands of hours of training the bodies of other people into this book.

Don't worry: this isn't an autobiography in which I wax lyrical about the celebrities and Premier League footballers I've trained. Yes, I have trained those types of people, but to me every client has the same goal for every training session: they want to get maximum results from the time they are prepared to invest in exercise. Every exercise I select for their session, therefore, has to have earned its place in the programme and every teaching point that I provide needs to be worthwhile and have a positive outcome. In essence, my teaching style could almost be described as minimalist. Now that the fitness industry enters its fourth decade, many of you will have accumulated a level of knowledge and information equal to some fitness professionals in the industry, so I don't go in for trying to show you how clever I am when all that is required are clear and concise instructions.

I learned this lesson many years ago when I was hired as personal trainer to a professor of medicine. There was absolutely nothing I could say about the function of the body that she didn't already know, but what I could do was assess her current level of ability and take her on the shortest, safest and most effective route to an improved level of fitness. Seventeen years on I am still finding new ways to help her enjoy and benefit from the time we spend training together.

The thought process and methods I use are based on my belief that every-body feels better when they build activity into their lives, but not everybody has the motivation and time to create the type of bodies we see on the covers of fitness magazines. When training my clients, I am ultimately judged on the results I deliver. These results can present themselves in many ways, for example, in the mirror or on the weighing scales, but I also aim to help my clients make sense of what we are doing together. I find when talking about any activity it is best to focus on the outcomes rather than use subjective classifications, such as beginner/advanced, easy/hard. Therefore, to help you make sense of each activity you'll be doing with the kettlebell, and how it relates to my S.A.F.E. training system, each move is classified by its respective outcome, whether that be an increase in stability, strength or power, rather than the more subjective easy, medium and hard.

every body is different

Just to be clear, any attempt to classify physical activity has to respect the fact that each human body responds to physical demands differently – there isn't an exact point where one move stops being beneficial for stability and switches over to being purely for strength. The transition is far more subtle and means that no matter which version of a move you are doing, you will never be wasting your time.

don't skip the moves

Human nature might lead you to think that the way to achieve the quickest results would be to skip the 'easy' stability and strength moves and start on day one with the power versions. Overcoming this instinct is fundamental for banishing the 'old school approach' of beating up the body every training session, rather than using your training time wisely. My approach is about quality and not quantity. For a personal trainer to take this approach it requires true confidence and belief in the system, as some clients (particularly men) feel that they should be 'working hard' every session. This, I feel, is a situation unique to fitness training. In no other sport or activity would you set out to teach the body to cope with a new skill or level of intensity by starting with the high intensity or fastest version. For example, if you are learning to play golf, you don't start by trying to hit the ball a long way – rather you start by simply trying to make contact and hit it in the right direction. Or how about tennis? When learning to serve, if all you do is hit the ball as hard as you can, it is unlikely that any shot will ever stay within the lines of the court and therefore count. I know this from personal experience as after many years fearlessly riding mountain bikes I have just taken up road racing and adapting my upright off-road skill to the very different requirements of adopting an aerodynamic position on a road bike. It required me to start slowly with the basics and progressively add speed when my skills had developed enough to be instinctive rather than challenged. In all cases, quality and the development of skill is the key to success rather than hoping that beating yourself up will turn out OK.

mixing it up

The sudden popularity of kettlebell usage has required experienced personal trainers to yet again think about human movement in a completely new way, especially when associated with the most overused word in the world of fitness – 'functional'. This description is often being used to describe exercise that has a direct relationship with the way we move in everyday life or during sporting activities. However, the types of challenges and forces that kettlebells inflict upon our bodies actually don't occur that often in everyday life. Therefore, you could question if kettlebells should be described as functional when, in fact, they are extreme, rather than everyday.

In just one decade the trend has gone from doing much of our strength training on machines that moved in straight lines to trying to incorporate the body's three planes of motion (sagittal, frontal and transverse) into all our conditioning exercises by using both improved weight machines and of course the huge selection of functional training products now available: sagittal involves movements from left to right of the body's centre line; frontal (coronal) involves movements which are forward and backward from the centre line and transverse which are movements that involve rotation. The reality is these planes of motion never occur independently of each other so the best way to ensure you are working through all three planes is to create exercises that incorporate bending and twisting rather than to look at joint movements in isolation.

Before the fitness industry started to think with a 'functional' mindset, it wasn't unusual to discourage any type of twisting during a workout; the introduction of

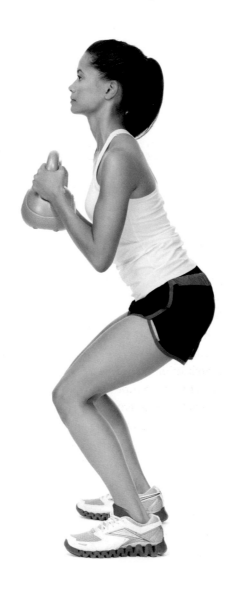

functional training equipment and in particular the popularity of the extremely dynamic kettlebell activities has evoked a completely different approach where we now actively look for ways to incorporate all the planes of motion into everything we do. The multi-plane moves don't altogether replace isolation moves that still have an important role to play (particularly if you are trying to overload and bulk up individual muscles). These isolation moves are generally good for overloading and challenging an individual muscle to adapt and react to the challenges of exercise, but working muscles one at a time leaves you with a body full of great individual muscle when what you actually need are muscles that work as a team and in conjunction with other muscles that surround them. For example, despite most of the classic free weight exercises being integrated movements (i.e. they work more than one set of muscles at a time), the vast majority of free weight moves involve no rotation of the spine (through the transverse plane) and therefore don't train the body for the reality of every day, where we constantly rotate at the same time as bending, pushing or pulling against external forces. Working muscles one at a time is not what a kettlebell session sets out to do; if that was the case, you would be better off using dumbbells and barbells.

Even when we do aim to target smaller groups of muscles rather than the body as a whole, the dynamic action of the unique swinging kettlebell moves enables them to be 'functional' rather than isolated, because in addition to the muscles being intentionally targeted, the moves have the additional benefit of directing force through the spine and lumbopelvic region and therefore activating the core stabilisers in a way that wouldn't occur if the same muscles were worked minus the build up of kinetic energy that the swing generates.

I can honestly say that until the late 1990s not a second thought was given to the muscles that we now refer to as 'core stabilisers'. There still seems to be a lack of understanding of how we can train the various components that go to create stabilisation of the spine and pelvis (muscle, ligaments, tendons and fascia). To put it simply, core stabilisation is a reaction that occurs when the body senses a need to maintain a position or to reposition itself urgently – the key word in there is 'reaction'. The core isn't permanently switched on but it is permanently primed and ready for action so next time you hear an exercise teacher tell you to 'switch on your core', you'll know they are wasting their breath unless there is some kind of physical challenge to make the body spring into action.

the workouts
In the final section of the book you will find a series of workouts. They are designed to be realistic sessions that you can do on any day of the week, without the need for 'rest' days or anything more than a reasonable amount of space.

All the workouts are sequential, so in theory you could start with 15 minutes of stability moves and do every workout until you reach 30 minutes of power moves. This is, of course, the theory; in reality you will naturally find the right start point depending on how you do with the assessment (see 'Assess, don't guess' on page 23) and how much time you have available on a given day. Continue using that particular workout until you feel ready to move on. I would advise everybody to start with the stability sessions, then move onto strength and then finally power, but I also accept that some people will find that the stability and strength moves don't challenge them enough so they will dive into the power phase. Please bear in mind that, if this is how you plan on approaching the exercises in this book, you might be missing out on a valuable learning curve that the body would benefit from.

a resource for life

My aim is for this book to be an ongoing reference point, and I suggest reading the entire contents and then dipping into the specific areas that interest you, such as the training programmes or fitness glossary. I guarantee you'll discover nuggets of information that perhaps you knew a little about, but had never fully understood because they had been explained in such a way that left you confused. If fitness training is an important part of your life, or even your career, then I know this book will be a long-term resource and will help you get the most from the time you spend using your equipment.

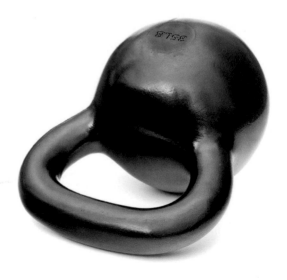

FAQs

When learning to train with kettlebells, there are a handful of important questions that you should ask before attempting to lift the weights. Find the answers here.

These are the most common questions that fitness trainers are asked in relation to exercising with a kettlebells.

Surely a weight is a weight so what's the difference in lifting a 12kg dumbbell and a 12kg kettlebell?

Yes, as far as gravity is concerned 12kg is 12kg when it is being dropped, but in a piece of fitness equipment the way that the weight (mass) is distributed makes a huge difference. In a dumbbell the weight is split between the two ends of the handle and is inline and close to the grip (handle), but in a kettlebell the mass is all in the ball section of the product. How far away from the handle this mass is positioned depends upon the specific design of the kettlebell. So, to put it simply, the further you move the weight away from the handle, the greater the effect you will experience when you swing the kettlebell.

Does the design of the kettlebell affect its performance?

Yes, as with all items of fitness equipment, you get what you pay for. The very cheapest weights can have handles that are at best uncomfortable to use and at worst potentially dangerous. When cheap raw materials are used (called pig iron), the horns of the handles have to be made extra thick and short to stop them from snapping when dropped. The shortness of the horns means that when you hold the kettlebell in the 'rack' position (resting on the back of your forearm) it is close to the wrist joint and therefore exerts unfavourable pressure on the joint and hits it directly when the weight is spun in the hand. A good quality, well-designed weight will have a distance of at least 5cm between the handle and the ball section of the kettlebell. Most gyms will be equipped with cast iron or steel kettlebells ranging from 8 to 32kg. If the kettlebells all vary in size, then they are 'classic' kettlebells but if they are all the same size irrespective of what weight they are, then they are probably what's classed as being 'competition' or 'pro grade'. This means that no matter what weight you are lifting, the dimensions of the weights are all the same. This is important to people who enter lifting competitions because they can develop their technique using the standard shape and not have to re-learn or change their methods as they progress to heavier weights. To help you identify the different weights competition kettlebells are colour coded: 8kg = Pink, 12kg = Blue, 16kg = Yellow, 20kg = Purple, 24kg = Green, 28kg = Orange and 32kg = Red. The pro grade kettlebells also have slimmer smoother handles which help to minimise fatigue in your grip when performing high repetition sets.

Do I need a pair of the same weight kettlebells to use this book or can I do the exercises with just one kettlebell?

From experience I know that many people only buy single kettlebells rather than pairs so I have selected the exercises so that you can perform them one side at a time. Physically lifting two weights is harder than lifting just one simply because of the cumulative weight but with kettlebell training the overriding influence is the speed at which you swing the kettlebell rather than aiming to lift bigger and bigger weights.

What weight kettlebells should I buy?

You may be surprised how quickly you progress up the weight range. In my experience women, who often start with less than 8kg, very quickly realise that they can use heavier weights up to 16kg once they have become accustomed to the techniques. For men, 12kg is a common starting point which quickly

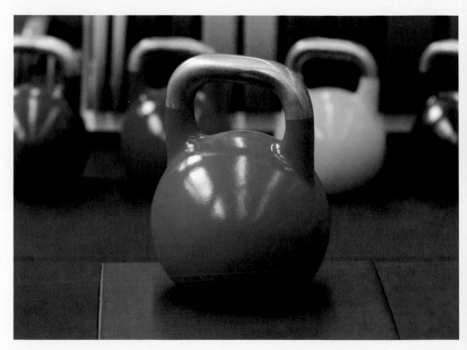

progresses to weights in the 16–24kg range. There are also adjustable kettlebells available which let you change the weight. Due to the way these are designed, the key point to remember is to ensure that the removable discs are fitted firmly together otherwise they will rattle when in use.

Does using a kettlebell create better results than using dumbbells and, if so, why?

Yes and no. A kettlebell can be used for many exercises usually performed with a dumbbell – moves such as bicep curls, shoulder press, squats and lunges rely on the addition of a dead weight to enhance their effectiveness or challenge of the movement. The unique characteristics of a kettlebell don't really come in to force, however, until there is speed or more specifically inertia included in the movement of the weight. The displaced mass of the kettlebell (i.e. the weight set away from the handle) causes reaction in the body that adds to the exercise by increasing muscle action, the amount of muscles actively recruited and exertion levels.

I have seen people doing kettlebell training with bare feet – why is this?

It's not just during kettlebell training that this is happening, many people are forgoing shoes during activities like running, pilates and yoga. The reason for this is a feeling that wearing training shoes de-activates or de-sensitises the muscles in the feet and the lower leg. Personally I agree with a lot of the studies on this, however, in reality unless you are an athlete who is looking for 1–5% improvement then the effects will be negligible.

What is 'core training'?

This subject can get very confusing so I thought it might help if I gave you my one-line description of what I think core training is.

Core training is: 'Exercise that develops strength and endurance for all muscles that protect the spine from damage and that function to produce dynamic movements'.

Or, the even shorter version: 'Exercise that makes you better at dealing with forces applied to the lumbopelvic region'.

As core training has evolved from physical therapy, where the main aim is to fix problems rather than achieve traditional fitness or cosmetic outcomes, there is a tendency to medicalise the subject. However, since my aim is to increase fitness rather than rehabilitation I approach core training with the same attitude as I do all of my training: you need to walk before you can run. Therefore, if I find that a person is having issues with their balance, stability and overall quality of movement, I start right from the beginning using the ball to re-train them to use (help activate) muscles and maintain postures at the lowest of intensity before moving on to what they would consider to be a 'workout'. But unlike many personal trainers who seem to revel in finding things wrong with their clients, I do not believe that everybody is bound to be broken in some way if they have not previously done 'core training'. Therefore, if you are healthy and injury free working the core does not need to feel like a visit to the doctor; it can and should be challenging and progressive but, above all, simple.

What are the core muscles?

The lumbopelvic region consists of the deep torso muscles, transversus abdominis, multifidus, internal obliques and the layers of muscle and fascia that make up the pelvic floor. These are key to the active support of the lumbar spine, but unfortunately they are also the most vulnerable to injury if neglected. Using any kind of functional training equipment or methods to encourage the recruitment of these muscles is productive because the muscle activity is involuntary so, rather than having to tell the body to do something, it simply gets on with the work that is required. In fact, these muscles are recruited a split second before any movements of the limbs, which suggests that they actually anticipate the force that will soon be going through the lumbar spine. Kettlebell training is perhaps the most aggressive method of challenging the core muscles but also one of the most effective.

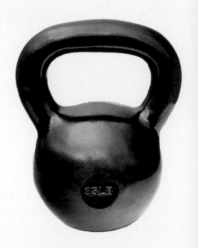

find your starting point

Before starting any exercise programme, test your body against the fitness checklist: mobility, flexibility, muscle recruitment and strength.

Before you think about doing any new type of exercise you need to establish what your starting point is, i.e. your current level of fitness, mobility, flexibility and strength. This is particularly important with kettlebells due to the dynamic nature of the activity. Every first consultation with a new personal training client revolves around the wish list of goals they hope to achieve. This list inevitably combines realistic goals with entirely unrealistic aims. Invariably people focus on their 'wants' rather than their 'needs' when goal-setting, and there is a big difference between the two mindsets. While 'wanting' could be considered a positive attitude, it will never overcome the need to slowly expose the body to processes that will change its characteristics and ability. Men in particular want to dive in at the most advanced stage of training, but it makes no sense to overload a muscle if your quality of movement is lacking.

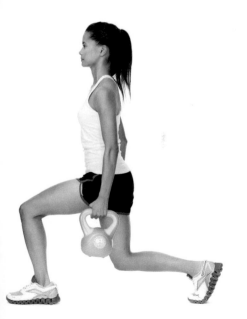
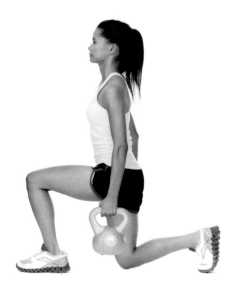

realiſtic goal-ſetting

The secret of realistic goal-setting is understanding the difference between these two words:

Want (v) 'A desired outcome'
Need (n) 'Circumstances requiring some course of action'

By identifying your needs, your goals may not sound so spectacular but you are more likely to achieve better and longer term results, and your progress through the fitness process will be considerably more productive. Therefore, rather than thinking about the ultimate outcome, think instead of resolutions to the 'issues'.

fitness checklist

The checklist you need to put your body through before you start swinging a kettlebell around is very simple and logical. Our ability to lift or move weight (by which I mean bodyweight as well as external loads) relies on a combination of:

- Mobility
- Flexibility
- Muscle recruitment
- Strength

If any of these vital components are neglected, it will have a knock-on effect on your progress. For example, while you may have the raw strength in your quadriceps to squat with a heavy weight, if you do not have a full range of motion in the ankle joints and sufficient flexibility in the calf muscles, then your squat will inevitably be of poor quality. Likewise, in gyms it is common to see men who have overtrained their chest muscles to such an extent that they can no longer achieve scapular retraction (they are round shouldered and therefore demonstrate poor technique in moves that require them to raise their arms above their heads).

This type of checklist is traditionally the most overlooked component of strength training and, while testing weight, body-fat levels and cardiac performance is now a regular occurrence in the fitness industry, the introduction of screening for quality of movement has taken a much longer time to become a priority, despite a self-administered assessment being as simple as looking in the mirror.

assess, don't guess

There is no better summary of the importance of our ability to move freely than in one of my favourite sayings: 'Use it or lose it'. This says it all – if you don't use the body to perform physical tasks it will more likely deteriorate than just stay the same.

It may be no coincidence that assessing movement quality has grown in importance for athletes and fitness enthusiasts at the same pace as the popularity of functional training – rightly so, because if you don't assess yourself, then how can you know what areas of functionality you need to work on most? Before functional training became a key component of progressive fitness programmes all progression related to increasing duration and intensity and resistance, whereas, now the quality of movement has become of equal importance.

Today, the assessment of 'functional movement', or biomechanical screening, is its own specialised industry within the world of fitness. Those working in orthopaedics and conventional medical rehabilitation have always followed some form of standardised assessment where they test the function of the nerves, muscles and bones before forming an opinion of a patient's condition. Becoming a trained practitioner takes many years of study and practice. Not only must a practitioner gain knowledge of a wide spectrum of potential conditions, but just as importantly they must understand when and how to treat their patient, or when they need to refer them to other colleagues in the medical profession. Having been subjected to and taught many different approaches to movement screening, in my mind, the challenge isn't establishing there is something 'wrong', but knowing what to do to rectify the issue.

mobility and flexibility

The most common problem limiting quality of movement in the average person is a lack of mobility and flexibility, which can be provisionally tested using the standing twist and the overhead squat assessment (see pages 25–26).

To understand why mobility is key to human movement, think how, as babies, we start to move independently. We are born with mobility and flexibility then we progressively develop stability, balance and then increasing levels of strength. As we get older we may experience injuries, periods of inactivity and, to some extent, stress, which all contribute towards a progressive reduction of mobility. There is no better summary of the importance of mobility than in one of my favourite

. . . .

sayings: 'Use it or lose it'. If you sit for extended periods or fail to move through the three planes of motion (see page 150), then you invariably become restricted in your motion. With this in mind, I hope you can see that lifting weights without first addressing mobility issues is like trying to build the walls of a house before you have completed the foundations.

The following two mobility tests challenge the entire length of the kinetic chain (actions and reactions to forces that occur in the bones, muscles and nerves whenever dynamic motion or force is required from the body) and help to reveal if you are ready to move beyond bodyweight moves to begin adding the additional loads such as kettlebells. This test focuses on the key areas of the shoulders, the mid-thoracic spine, the pelvis, the knees, ankles and feet. Any limitation of mobility, flexibility or strength in these areas will show up as either an inability to move smoothly through the exercise or an inability to hold the body in the desired position.

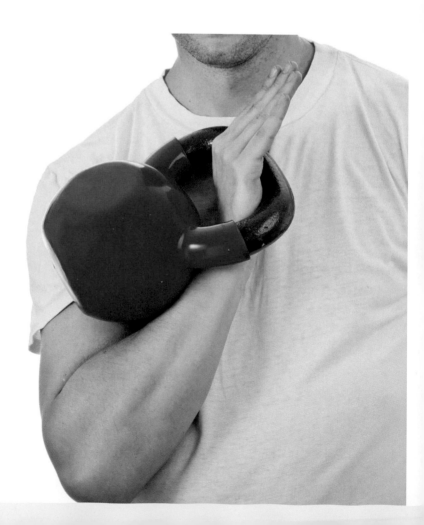

Test 1 standing twist

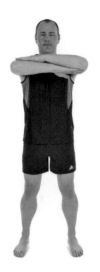 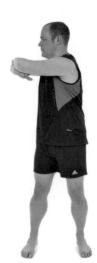

This is the less dramatic of the two mobility tests and serves to highlight if you have any pain that only presents when you move through the outer regions of your range of movement, and also if you have a similar range of motion between rotations on the left and right sides of your body.

- Stand with your feet beneath your hips.
- Raise your arms to chest height then rotate as far as you can to the right, noting how far you can twist.
- Repeat the movement to the left.
- Perform the movement slowly so that no 'extra twist' is achieved using speed and momentum.

You are trying to identify any pain and/or restriction of movement. If you find either, it might be the case that this reduces after a warm-up or a few additional repetitions of this particular movement. If you continue to experience pain, you should consider having it assessed by a physiotherapist or sports therapist.

Test 2 overhead squat (OHS)

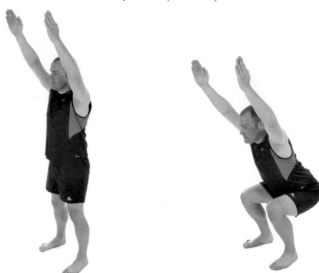

I've used the OHS test over 5000 times as part of my S.A.F.E. approach to exercise and I have found it to be the quickest and easiest way of looking at basic joint and muscle function without getting drawn into speculative diagnosis of what is and isn't working properly. If you can perform this move without any pain or restriction, you will find most of the moves in this book achievable. There is no pass or fail; rather you will fall into one of two categories: 'good' or 'could do better'. If you cannot achieve any of the key requirements of the OHS move, then it is your body's way of flagging up that you are tight and/or weak in that particular area. This, in turn, could mean you have an imbalance, pain or an untreated injury, which may not prevent you from exercising, but which you should probably get checked out by a physiotherapist or sports therapist.

Perform this exercise barefoot and in front of a full-length mirror so that you can gain maximum information from the observation of your whole body. Also refer to Table 1 for a list of key body regions to observe during this test. (This move also doubles up as a brilliant warm-up for many types of exercise including lifting weights.)

- Stand with feet pointing straight ahead and at hip width.
- Have your hands in the 'thumbs-up position' and raise your arms above your head, keeping them straight, into the top of a 'Y' position (with your body being the bottom of the 'Y'). Your arms are in the correct position when they are back far enough to disappear from your peripheral vision.

- The squat down is slow and deep, so take a slow count of six to get down by bending your knees. The reason we go slowly is so you do not allow gravity to take over and merely slump down. Also, by going slowly you get a chance to see and feel how everything is moving through the six key areas.

The magic of this move is that you will be able to see and feel where your problem spots are and, even better, the test becomes the solution, because simply performing it regularly helps with your quality of movement. Stretch out any area that feels tight and aim to work any area that feels weak.

Table 1 Key body regions to observe in the overhead squat

Body region	Good position	Bad position
Neck		
Shoulders		
Mid-thoracic spine		
Hips		

Body region	Good position	Bad position
Knees		
Ankles and feet		

As you perform the OHS you are looking for control and symmetry throughout and certain key indicators that all is well:

- **Neck:** You keep good control over your head movements and are able to maintain the arm lift without pain in the neck.
- **Shoulders:** In the start position and throughout the move you are aiming to have both arms lifted above the head and retracted enough so that they are outside your peripheral vision (especially when you are in the deep part of the squat). In addition to observing the shoulders, look up at your arms to the hands – throughout the OHS you should aim to have your thumbs pointing behind you.
- **Mid-thoracic spine:** There is no instruction to keep your back straight, so in this area of the body you are looking for 'flow' rather than clunking movements.
- **Hips:** Imagine a straight line drawn directly down the centre of your body. Around the hips you are looking to see if you shift your weight habitually to one side, rather than keeping it evenly spread between both sides.
- **Knees:** The most common observation is the knees touching during the OHS, suggesting a weakness in the glutes. Less common is the knees parting, showing weakness in the inner thigh. Good technique is when your knees move forwards as you bend the legs. Note that clicking and crunching noises don't always suggest a problem unless they are accompanied by pain.
- **Ankles and feet:** The most obvious issue is the heels lifting from the floor, suggesting short achilles and calf muscles. Less obvious are the flattening of the

foot arches that cause the feet to roll inward (overpronation) or the foot rolling outward (underpronation). Ideally, the foot should be in a neutral position.

If, when you do the OHS in front of the mirror, you observe any of these signals with your kinetic chain (the actions and reactions to forces that occur in the bones, muscles and nerves whenever dynamic motion or force is required from the body), it really isn't the end of the world. In fact, most people find that they are tight in some areas (if not all of them) when they first try this test. The absolutely fantastic news is that if you do spot any issues, performing the OHS as an exercise, rather than merely a test, will improve your movement pattern, joint range and muscle actions over time.

overhead squat: the results

My rule is that if you cannot perform a perfect OHS, with none of the key warning signs listed above, then you are not ready to perform the power moves in the exercise portfolio. So use the OHS as a guide to whether your body is as ready as your mind is to start doing the toughest, most challenging exercises.

If you find by doing the OHS that your body is not ready, don't think of it as a setback, but rather as a blessing: you are following a training method that is in tune with how the body works, rather than one that merely sets out to punish it.

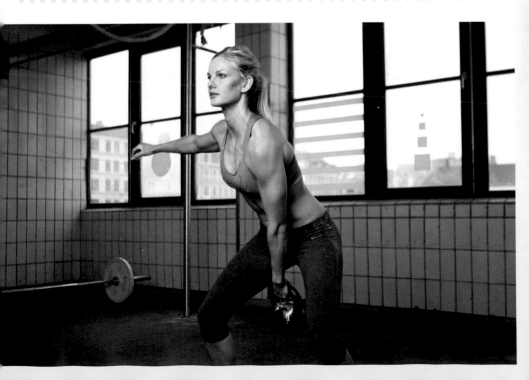

isolation vs integration

While intensity can be great, when you isolate your muscles you do not get the highly beneficial activity created by the rest of the kinetic chain. I am certainly not saying isolation moves are unproductive, but with the biggest obstacle to exercise being a lack of time, integration work is going to have an instant usable impact on the entire body.

All movements that we do in training or everyday life can be classified as either isolation or integration moves. The vast majority of isolation moves have been created/invented to work specific muscles on their own, with the primary intention of fatiguing that muscle by working it in isolation, usually moving only one joint of the skeleton. Integration, or compound, moves are less of an invention and more of an adaptation of movement patterns that we perform in everyday life. They are designed to work groups of muscles across multiple joints all at the same time.

In real life we never isolate. Even when only a few joints are moving there is a massive number of muscles bracing throughout the body to let the prime muscles do their job. As you go about an average day I doubt you give a second thought to how you are moving. If you take the time to watch the world go by for a few hours, you will notice that human motion consists of just a few combinations of movements that, together, create the millions of potential moves we (hopefully) achieve every day. Everything, and I mean everything, we do boils down to the following key movements:

- Push
- Pull
- Twist
- Squat
- Lunge
- Bend
- Walk
- Run
- Jump

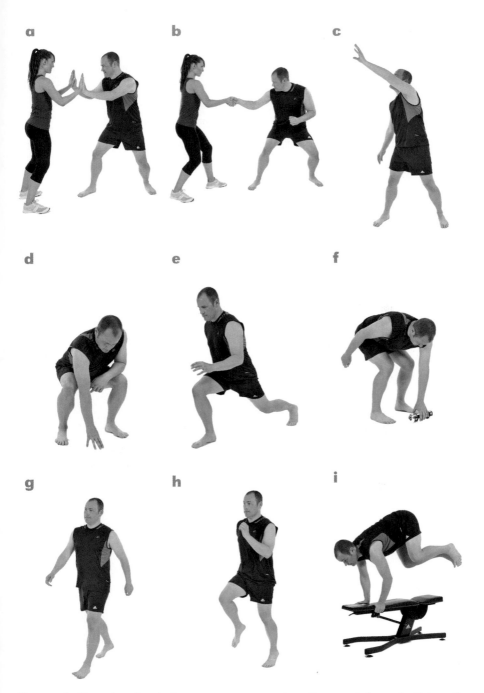

Figure 1 The nine basic human movement patterns: (a) push, (b) pull, (c) twist, (d) squat, (e) lunge, (f) bend, (g) walk, (h) run and (i) jump

All of these movements are integrated. I am certainly not the first person to make this observation, but it constantly amazes me how my industry manages to complicate exercise. With this in mind, I am not a huge fan of old-fashioned machines that isolate small areas of muscle to work them apparently more intensely. While intensity can be great, when you isolate you do not get the highly beneficial activity created by the rest of the kinetic chain. I am certainly not saying isolation moves are unproductive, but with the biggest obstacle to exercise being a lack of time, integration work is going to have an instant usable impact on the entire body.

We would rarely incorporate isolation moves into a workout with a kettlebell as this defeats the object of having a product which challenges the body as a whole. Even when a move is targeted towards smaller muscle groups such as the pecs or the triceps, it would still be considered to be an integration (compound) move because, the displaced mass of a kettlebell means that even a 'simple' exercise like a bicep curl directs force through the lumbopelvic region, which therefore also activates the core stabilisers. Consequently, the majority of the moves in this book are integrated, designed to achieve maximum results in the most economical amount of time.

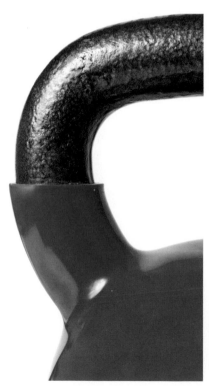

learn it, then work it

As we have discovered, you must walk before you can run in any exercise method, and the body works best if you learn the activity prior to engaging in exercise, so that you will positively soak up the benefits.

Resistance training (using either bodyweight or free weights, or both) is very natural with hardly any complex skills required to achieve results. However, that is not to say you can't get it wrong. In fact, re-building the confidence of people who have tried weight training and then failed or injured themselves has featured frequently in my working life. Because of this, I use the phrase 'learn it, then work it' to encourage people to take time to 'imprint' good-quality movement patterns upon their bodies.

how to 'learn it, then work it'

How do you know what 'good quality' moves look like? Simply put, the move should look smooth and controlled and should not create pain in your joints. Aim to perform the concentric and eccentric phases (the lift and lower phases) at the same speed – lift for two counts and lower for two counts. When power and speed become more of an objective for you, aim to lift for one count and lower for two counts.

You can perform moves at slower speeds, but that then moves away from how we move/function in day-to-day life; rarely do we do any movement in slow motion just for the sake of it. It is really only beneficial to perform slow or super slow (quarter-speed) moves if you are training for specific sport activities, so as to prolong the time each muscle is under tension (known as 'time under tension'). Therefore, move at a natural speed: athletes and sports people train at 'real time' once they have learned the required movement pattern, so without even knowing it they are 'learning it, then working it'.

The beauty of grounding your workout in the 'learn it, then work it' approach is that by keeping the approach simple, achievable and functional you won't get tied up with methods that either do not work, or have ridiculous expectations of how much time you are going to dedicate to your fitness regime. As a personal trainer, it can be hard to exercise in a gymnasium without wanting to question what many people are (or think they are) doing. So often I see people doing difficult versions of exercises that are clearly beyond their level of ability – presumably because they think difficult/advanced must equal quicker results. The obvious signs are that they can't control the weights or their body seems overpowered by the movements it is being asked to do. 'Learn it, then work it' relates to most physical tasks in life, but especially sport; for example, if you have tennis lessons, the first thing you would learn would be to make contact with the ball slowly rather than starting with the fastest, hardest movements. So simply switch off your instincts to 'work hard' until you are satisfied that you can move and maintain quality and control throughout the repetition.

As you get more adventurous and diverse with your exercise remember that all your goals are achievable: if you're moving, you're improving.

'learn it, then work it' in sport

Practising movements in resistance training is paralleled in all performance-based sports. Athletes routinely perform low intensity 'drills', which echo the moves they need to make in their sport. For example, during almost every track session, sprinters practise knee lifts, heel flicks and other bounding exercises to improve their quality of movement and condition their muscles in a highly functional manner.

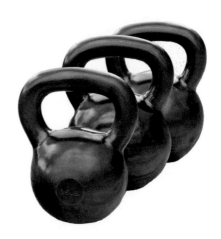

first you need stability

Stability is the first key ingredient to ensure safe and effective exercise; the basic building block for everything that follows in this book.

To perform exercise safely and effectively, we first have to ensure our body is stable. The essence of stability is the ability to control and transfer force throughout the body. All human movement is, in fact, a chain of events involving the brain, the nervous system, muscles, fascia, ligaments and tendons. So, while a simple move like a bicep curl may appear to involve only activity from the shoulder down to the hand, in reality there is a chain of events that occur to ensure that the right amount of force is applied and that the two ends of the bicep are tethered to a stable base.

In essence, wherever there is visible movement in the body, there are always invisible reactions occurring within the kinetic chain to facilitate this movement.

The engine room of all this activity is in the deep muscles of the trunk, specifically:

- transversus abdominus (TA);
- multifidi (MF);
- internal obliques;
- five layers of muscle and fascia that make up the pelvic floor.

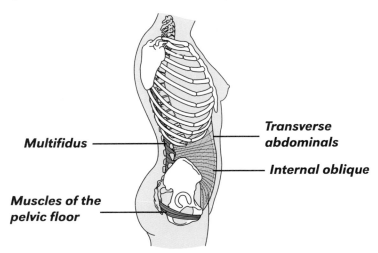

Figure 2 The deep muscles of the trunk are crucial for stability

These muscles work as a team and their simultaneous contraction is known as 'co-contraction'. This complex muscle activity produces intra-abdominal pressure (IAP) and it is the creation of this pressure that stabilises the lumbar spine. The misconception that the transversus abdominus looks like a 'belt' around the torso no doubt led fitness instructors to continually advise clients to pull their stomach in (hollow the abdominal muscles), thinking that this would amplify the stability of the spine. However, it is not simply the recruitment of these muscles that instils strength and stability, but, more importantly, when they are recruited. In effect, they should have been advising clients to 'switch on' (brace their core).

remember: don't hollow your abs

Pulling in, or hollowing, the abs actually makes you less able to stabilise. If you imagine a tree that is perfectly vertical, but then you chop in or hollow out one side, the structure of the tree becomes less stable. I have two ways of coaching the correct technique to avoid hollowing the abs, depending on the client:

1 Switch on your abs as if you were going to get punched in the stomach, or
2 Engage the abs in the same way as if you were about to be tickled.

Both methods achieve the desired outcome – with only a few of my male clients insisting that I really do hit them!

Stability is, therefore, a goal in everything that we do. However, we shouldn't have to undertake yet more training just to achieve core stability; rather, we should ensure that the everyday movements we make encourage the muscles deep inside the trunk to work correctly during dynamic movements, and that the stabilisation is instinctive, as opposed to something that we have to remind ourselves to do every time. For instance, if you drop an egg in the kitchen and very quickly squat and make a grab to catch it, you don't stop to think or choreograph the movement. Your body will have fired off a co-contraction which enabled you to grab the egg before it hit the ground (or, at least, make a good attempt). When I use this analogy to explain the concept of stability to my clients, they often get a twinkle in their eye, for if this process is instinctive, why should they continue to train? The reality, however, is that you still have to exercise that instinct to keep the system working properly: 'use it, or lose it'.

In the workout sessions later in this book, you will find that almost all the moves are classified as being good for stability. Since stability is the first stage of development, you might assume the strength and power moves that follow are more productive because they are more 'intense'. While this is true, that intensity will only be constructive if the body has the ability to control and direct all that extra force, which can only be learned through the stability moves.

the development of core stability in the fitness industry

During the 1990s, there were only three components of fitness that personal trainers focused on with the average client (by 'average' I mean a person looking for fitness gains rather than to compete in sport). Cardio was the route to cardiovascular efficiency and was the most obvious tool for weight loss; strength training isolated the larger muscle groups and gymnasiums were filled with straight line machines; and we only worked on flexibility because we knew we had to, but the chosen method was predominantly the least productive type of stretching, i.e. static.

Then, it seems almost from nowhere, there was a new ingredient to every workout: core stability. New equipment such as Swiss balls and modern versions of wobble boards, such as the Reebok Core Board® and the BOSU® (Both Sides Up), increased the wave of enthusiasm for this type of training as, of course, did the new popularity for the more physical versions of yoga and Pilates.

In retrospect, we in the fitness industry could have thought to ourselves that we had been doing everything wrong up to that point. However, the reality is that rather than being 'wrong' we were just learning as we went along. In fact, many of the methods that suddenly became mainstream had been used in sports training for years before, but without the 'label' of core stability, and rather than treating them as an individual component, we trained them instinctively as part of our dynamic strength moves using bodyweight or free weights.

add some strength

The second key ingredient. There are several types of strength that you can gain performing these exercises with kettlebells (dynamic and static).

When trying to establish a client's fitness objectives, 'I want to improve my strength' is often the only information given to a personal trainer. This seemingly simple request requires much more detail if you are going to achieve the outcome that is really desired.

The one-line definition of strength is: 'An ability to exert a physical force against resistance'. However, this catch-all is not specific enough when you are dealing with strength. In fact, there are three main types of strength:

1 **Strength endurance:** Achieved when you aim to exert force many times in close succession.
2 **Elastic strength:** Achieved when you make fast contractions to change position.
3 **Maximum strength:** Our ability over a single repetition to generate our greatest amount of force.

Each of these specific types of strength can be achieved using resistance, either as individual components or (preferably) as part of an integrated approach.

Unless you are an athlete training for an event that requires a disproportionate amount of either endurance, elastic or maximum strength, then the integration of functional training methods will create a body that is more designed to cope with day-to-day life and amateur sports. While strength is an adaptation that the body willingly accepts, the reality is that changes take time, so treat strength gains as something that happens over weeks, months and years rather than mere days.

power and speed come with practice

The development of power in muscles is a rapid process and is also considerably practical, usable and functional for those men and women who have reached a point in their training where they don't need to be any 'stronger', but they want to make more of the strength they have.

Power is a measure of how much energy is created, the amount of force applied and the velocity at which it is applied. It is the ability to exert an explosive burst of movement. In everyday life it presents as bounding up stairs three at a time or pushing a heavy weight above your head. The development of power is not only a more rapid process than developing maximal strength, but is also considerably more practical, usable and functional for those men and women who have reached a point in their training where they have no desire to be any 'stronger', but they do want to make more of the strength they have. That is the point at which you stop thinking about increasing the amount of resistance you work against and start thinking about how to inject speed into the activity you are doing with the kettlebell and increasing the number of exercises that specifically include the swinging motion.

Let's make this simple. If you have two men of the same height, weight and with the same body fat levels and you challenge them to compete against each other in an explosive activity that they have both trained in, such as a 20m sprint, then, apart from potential differences in reaction times, the man who wins that race will be the one who has a greater ability to utilise his strength and convert that strength into forward motion. This ability to use strength for explosive activity is power. The perfect exercise to generate this type of outcome would be the squat against a wall with a jump as this move trains you to generate an explosive force that propels the body quickly.

When you get to the exercises in the portfolio classified as power moves, you will see that they are, in fact progressions of the skills that you will have already developed during your stability and strength sessions, but performed at speed. In this respect, it becomes easier to understand why I advise not to skip a stage when learning movement patterns ('learn it, then work it').

To train or develop power using predominately kettlebells is entirely logical, but only as long as you do not get preoccupied with the speed part of the equation to the detriment of working through the correct range of motion. It is very easy to 'cheat' with a kettlebell – cheating can be classed as not doing a full range of motion, shifting your bodyweight so that the exercise becomes easier – any of these 'cheating tactics' will allow you to move faster but you will probably not be using as much strength as you would without the adaptation.

power and agility

Think of power as a very close relation of agility; you don't learn agility by overloading and working while fatigued – rather you develop it by achieving quality over quantity. In fact, introducing yourself to the pursuit of power can mean performing the moves without any weights and simply performing the movements fast with just bodyweight as the resistance. Why? Because athletic power is actually a finely tuned combination of speed and strength.

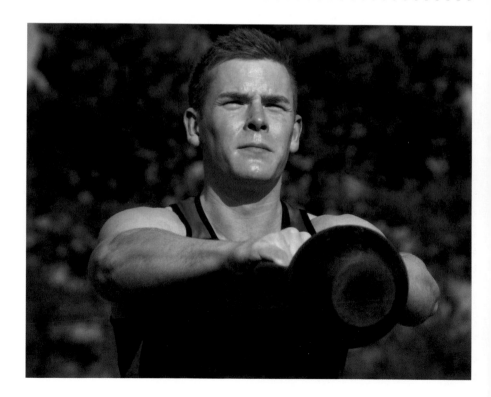

2 the portfolio of moves

which moves should I do?

This section contains a portfolio of moves that I have selected from those I use every day with my personal training clients and are based on the principles I explained in the first part of this book. The only moves that have made it into this book are those that deserve to be here – every one of these moves is tried and tested to ensure it gets results; in fact, I have spent hundreds of hours using them myself and thousands of hours teaching them to my personal training clients, who over the years have included men and women from 16 to 86 years old, from size zero through to 280lbs. These clients have, justifiably, only been interested in the moves that work – and those are what you have here in this portfolio.

It is not an exhaustive list of moves, simply because many extra moves that could have been included use the kettlebell simply as a 'prop' rather than a tool, or they are really just subtle adaptations of those already included here. For instance, changes to foot position and the amount of bend that you have in your arms and legs will encourage the body to recruit slightly different muscles, but I would class these as adaptations rather than unique moves. I've also excluded any moves which use the kettlebell as a balance tool on the floor, because for this to be safe your kettlebell has to have a smooth base which isn't always the case.

presentation of the moves

I wanted to show the moves as a complete portfolio, rather than simply wrapping them up into workouts, because you are then able to see how the stability, strength and power versions relate to each other. Understanding these progressions is something I encourage in my clients because they need to know that subtle changes can make all the difference between a good use of time and a waste of it. By thinking this way you can very quickly learn all the moves because, in the majority of cases, the main movement pattern stays the same throughout the stability, strength and power progressions, with only a slight change to the length of levers (arm/foot positions), range of motion or the speed.

exercises to avoid

I've included a section for reference of exercises that I don't recommend. Some of these are exercises I have seen being performed in gyms around the world that I think are simply dangerous – for example, a kettlebell hanging from the foot. Others either achieve very little or when deconstructed can be performed quicker and more effectively by doing other moves included in the exercise programs – the Turkish Get Up, for example, is really just a selection of exercises strung together rather than being just one move. Multiple moves are great but stringing moves together is merging into choreography rather than training. I've tried to explain why I'm not a fan of these moves and, to keep things positive, I've also included a suitable replacement move for each of these exercises.

The third part of this book then goes on to present a selection of training sessions, designed for a range of levels, and following my method of progressing through stability, strength and power exercises, no doubt some people will jump straight to the training sessions. However I find understanding the 'why' as well as knowing the 'how' generates better outcomes for most people, so refer back to the portfolio of moves if you want the detailed description of how to perform the exercise. I have also provided you with a post-workout stretch session suitable for all types of resistance training (see pages 118–121). Please remember that you should always warm up before embarking on any type of exercise.

every muscle plays a part

I purposefully haven't included diagrams of the muscles that are targeted by each move as hopefully by now you understand that, used correctly, every muscle plays a role in every move.

I have written the descriptions as if I am talking to you as a client – the key information for each explanation includes:

- the correct body position at the start and end of the move;
- the movement that you are looking to create.

When I work with my PT clients I avoid over-coaching the movement as my goal is to see them move in a lovely 'fluid' way, where the whole movement blends together.

reps

This is a 'learn it' section rather than 'work it'. Therefore, for the vast majority of the moves I don't talk about how many repetitions you should do of each – that information is included in the workout section in the third part of the book. How many repetitions you perform should relate to your objectives; almost all the moves can be used to improve stability, strength and power (at the same time), and the speed and resistance at which you perform it will dictate the outcome. For example, a slow squat performed with a light weight will provide stability benefits. Exactly the same move performed with a heavier weight will increase strength, and the same move at speed will develop power.

In the workout section I have opted to set time challenges rather than state how many reps I want simply because I wanted to vary the challenges and improve the outcomes for all users. With kettlebells the activity (time under tension) is continuous rather than 'stop start', so when it comes to just counting repetitions taller people are at a disadvantage, therefore, aiming to perform the moves for a total number of seconds rather than reps works best.

weight

As speed and resistance are both subjective (one person's 'light' is another person's 'heavy'), it is simply not possible to predict how strong you are without seeing you actually work out. Choosing the correct weight is a matter of common sense and experience, so without being in the same room as you and looking at how you move and your physical characteristics it is hard to say exactly how much you should be lifting. My advice is always this: start with a weight that you can control but is challenging. As you fatigue, lifting the weights will get harder and the last two repetitions of the set should be tough to do.

tricks of the trade

For each exercise, I have included a 'tricks of the trade' box which contains a nugget of information that I use to help my clients get the most out of each exercises. This might be a physical trick or a coping strategy that helps them get the best out of the move.

key to exercises

As you move through the exercises, you will notice that each is identified by the following key words. A quick glance will tell you which element the move focuses on, what type of move it is and whether you need any additional equipment to perform it.

stability

Every move in this portfolio is a stability-enhancing exercise. Yes, that includes the strength and power versions. Stability is, essentially, a reaction within the kinetic chain in which the body says to itself: 'Switch on the muscles around the lumbopelvic region, because this movement is looking for an anchor point to latch on to'. On this basis, you still improve stability when you are doing the non-'swinging' moves based on the fact that we perform all the moves in positions that I've selected to specifically promote the need to activate stabilisation, rather than avoid it.

strength

We could get all deep and meaningful about biomechanics here, but to qualify as a strength move, the exercise needs to be making you move a force through space using muscle contractions. Therefore, anything that only involves momentum is a waste of time because you are just going along for the ride and not actively contracting your muscles. However, don't confuse speed with momentum – speed is good, especially when mixed with strength, because that combination develops the highly desirable power.

power

Every time you read the word 'power' you need to think of speed, and vice versa. The maths and physics required to understand how we measure power are enough to make you glaze over, and in reality you are much better off measuring your power ability by doing a simple time-trial sprint, or timing yourself over a set number of repetitions, rather than trying to calculate exactly how much power you are exerting for a specific exercise.

If you want more power, you need to move fast, but you need to be able to maintain speed while pushing or pulling a weight (that weight could be an object or your own body). For example, you might have a guy who can skip across a shot put circle faster than the other guy when not holding and throwing the shot, but he is only speedy. The guy who can move fast and launch the shot (using strength) is the one with all the power.

technique and 'grips' for safety and effectiveness

grip

When holding a kettlebell with one hand, your grip is integral to you being able to move the kettlebell safely and comfortably. The size of the handle on your kettlebells will vary depending upon their weight and design, however, your hand position is the same no matter what size they are – a good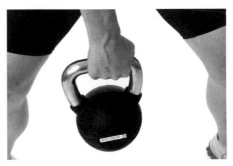
over-grip position has your hand positioned so that your thumb and index finger are towards the corner of where the handle meets the horns. You aren't trying to 'crush' the handle so while I wouldn't describe the grip as being 'relaxed', you should be able to let the handle rotate in your hand when you swing, clean or snatch.

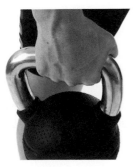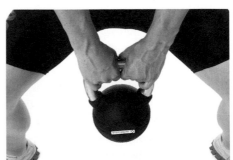

rack

For many kettlebell exercises the weight is positioned on the back of the arm. When the weight is positioned on there it is referred to as being in the 'rack' position. When you start using kettlebells getting from a swing into the rack position can be a shock as you have to develop and learn the ability to absorb (decelerate) the kettlebell as it comes to rest on your forearm. The most common mistake people make is having their wrist extended rather than in the neutral position – the extended wrist position is uncomfortable especially when the weight 'hits' the back of your wrist and it actually makes the kettlebell feel heavier. If you avoid the extended position, the kettlebell comes to rest on the back of the forearm less aggressively.

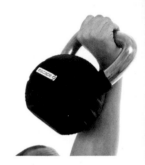

the Swing, Clean and Snatch

These are key movement patterns that are integrated into many of the classic kettlebell exercises so, along with good grip technique, learning and understanding these moves early on will help you to perform them better when they become part of your workout!

swing

The grip for the swing is also an over-grip. The first time you pick up a kettlebell, the temptation is to swing the kettlebell through your legs and hope for the best. This could either lead to at worst an injury or at least you scaring yourself! The better method is to be realistic about how much swing you can or should do first time. The best way I find to get clients ready to go for a full swing is to first practise with a 'restricted swing' – meaning that rather than dealing with the entire swing motion you only perform the bottom and middle part of the swing:

- Begin with the kettlebell hanging in front of you, bend your legs and start the weight swinging (the first swing just gets the weight moving).
- Keep your upper arm snug against your body rather than letting it be lifted up in front by the momentum of the kettlebell and hinge at the waist so the kettlebell goes through your legs. At this point the thumb on your gripping hand should be pointing upwards.

- Now drive the kettlebell forwards and up by using your legs and hips. When the kettlebell reaches shoulder height let it fall back through the legs and repeat.

With the kettlebell fixed in this restricted position the effort required is less than with a full swing and this means you can get used to the sensation of the swing rather than being overawed by the full blown swing.

clean

When lifting weights the 'clean' is what we call the technique for getting the weight from waist height up to chest/shoulder height. With barbells and dumbbells the weight travels up vertically, but with a kettlebell we need to incorporate some swing due the majority of the weight being offset from the handle.

The technique for the kettlebell swing is very different from the clean that you perform with a barbell. When using the kettlebell, the most important difference is that you keep your arms in tight to your torso. When working with clients I will sometimes use a band to hold their arms in to encourage them to get it right, but when working on your own just try to keep your triceps touching the sides of your ribs as much as possible.

- Start with a swing action driving back with your hips and legs. As the weight reaches chest height, allow the handle to slide in your hand so the ball of the kettlebell swings over the hand and comes to a rest on the back of your forearm.
- In this rack position, hold the weight in close to your body.
- Punch the weight away from you to start the swing action again and repeat.

snatch

The snatch is effectively a combination of a swing and clean combined into one smooth movement. The grip is a standard relaxed over-grip – this is important because you don't want to restrict the handle's ability to rotate in your hand. When performing a snatch it is a good idea to perform a couple of reps of the swing before you extend all the way through to have the kettlebell finishing above your head. You are trying to create enough energy from the swing to enable the kettlebell to swing all the way above you and gently come to a rest on the back of your forearm. The mistake many people make is to try to 'flick' the weight over at the top of the movement – this suggests they didn't generate enough force in the swing or that they performed the swing with a very bent arm which forces them to push up at the end of the swing rather than letting the kettlebell come to a controlled rest.

stretches

pre-exertion warm-up stretches

In previous decades we would stretch as part of our warm-up, but static stretching before exertion is now considered counter-productive as it inhibits some of your potential strength. It's very logical if you think about it, as stretching relaxes both mind and muscle! This is another example of how methods change throughout the years – it doesn't mean that we were wrong, just that our understanding of the body continues to evolve.

post-exertion stretches

Post exercise I have two different modes when I stretch:

1 If I am actively trying to increase my flexibility (stretch mode), I am going to take the position to the point of discomfort, hold it then keep going a little further. When the muscle relaxes, release the stretch for a moment then go back in to the stretch position again – the minimum time you should spend doing this is 30 seconds per stretch. There's no upper limit on how long you can stretch for, although it is essential that you do all the stretches equally rather than just focusing on the ones you enjoy or find easy.

2 When I am chilled out (relax mode), I just get into positions that are comfortable and enjoy the moment.

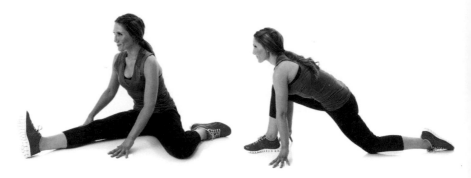

Modified hurdle stretch   **Hip stretch**

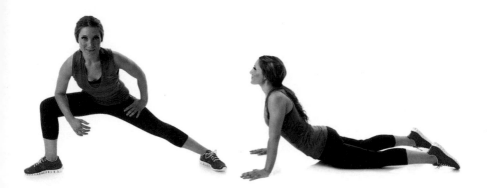

Inner thigh   **Back extension**

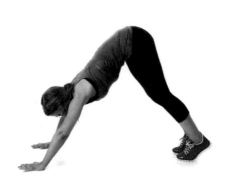

Down dog

dynamic warm-up moves

exercise 1 roll ups and downs

● **prepares body**

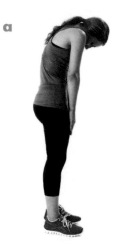

a

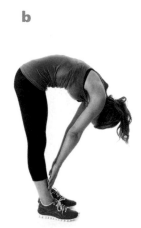

b

At first glance this exercise looks like you simply bend down and touch your toes, but the goal is mobilisation rather than flexibility. In fact if you can't touch your toes, you should forget all about swinging kettlebells around until you can. Using kettlebells are dynamic so 'body awareness' is very important – this move helps you to 'zone in' on the way your back moves.

● Keeping your hands close to your body, roll down towards the floor.
● Breathe out slowly as you lower.
● When/if your hands reach the floor, bend the knees, straighten again and stand up slowly.

tricks of the trade
As you bend forward, let your weight shift to the front of your feet and then as you stand up, shift the pressure back on to your heels and gently lift your head up at the top of the move. Shifting the weight will help to enhance your balance ready for the workout moves.

exercise 2 deep squat

• prepares body

a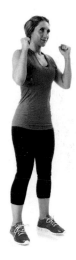

b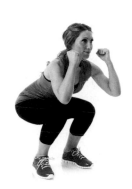

This movement is in reality much more of an essential move than an optional one. You can probably do this move already, however, it might require some time to perfect it because many misguided fitness instructors used to forbid clients to squat past 90 degrees at the knee. If it is 'too hard', try lying on your back and pulling both knees in to your chest – you'll prove to yourself that your hips and knees can flex enough – then stand up and do it properly.

- Stand with your feet at hip width apart. Looking ahead (not at the floor), squat down keeping your heels down.
- When you reach the lowest point, stand up with the emphasis on your glutes and hamstrings.

tricks of the trade
If depth is a problem, practise the move sliding up and down a wall with the aim of keeping your heels down.

exercise 3 hip hinges

• **prepares body**

 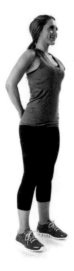

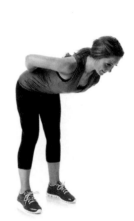

I can remember the first time I tried to do this move, it seemed so at odds with everything I had been doing previously. The aim is to 'brace' your torso by using your abdominal wall, but at the same time you will be going through a movement pattern that demands that you stabilise your pelvis while flexing – which makes this move fantastic and functional.

- Squeeze your shoulder blades together and bend forward.
- The temptation is to 'bow' from the waist but this movement initiates from the hips.
- Aim to create a 90 degree angle between your legs and back, then stand up slowly.

tricks of the trade
Controlling your breathing is a key part of this move: breathe out slowly on the way down and in on the way up.

exercise 4 heel reaches

• prepares body

a
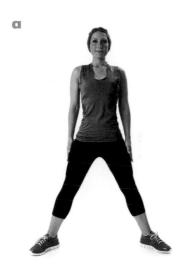

b
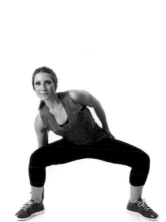

This move mixes things up. When we warm up the reality is it's the movement patterns that we avoid during our everyday life that we need to work on rather than simply repeating stuff that we are already good at. So the subtle difference between touching the toes and touching the heels is actually worlds apart, making the latter a fantastic exercise.

- Stand with your feet a little wider that your shoulders.
- Reach down the back of your leg with one hand, leaning down towards the foot on that side.
- Push back up and immediately repeat on the other side.

tricks of the trade
Start with small movements and build up the range of motion. You'll soon find you are reaching deeper.

exercise 5 dynamic shoulder swings

• **prepares body**

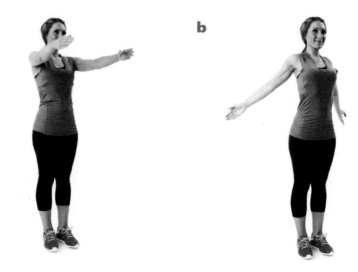

a

b

Apart from a direct impact (hit) on a muscle, the deceleration phase of dynamic movements is when all the soft tissue is most vulnerable to injury. By adding a kettlebell the acceleration and deceleration forces can be multiplied by three to four times so this move should be considered an essential warm-up for all kettlebell users.

- Place your feet closely together.
- Lift both arms in front of you and circle them backwards.
- Aim to feel the activity in the upper back and chest as well as the arm/shoulder joint.

tricks of the trade

Do more of these than you think you need to and make the circles big and slow rather than going fast. Also, remember to go in both directions to let the entire shoulder girdle warm up.

exercise 6 hip thrusters

 prepares body

a
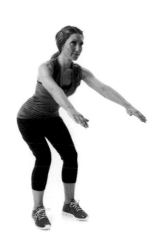

b
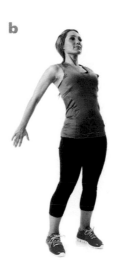

The number one 'school boy' error when doing kettlebell swings is lifting with the arms rather than getting the drive from the legs and hips. Following my mantra 'learn it, then work it', practising this move is therefore a 'must'. Yes, you might feel a bit stupid doing it in the gym, but that's better than getting injured!

- This move enhances muscle memory.
- Roll your shoulders forwards, with your arms in front.
- Drive the hips forwards and simultaneously swing your arms backwards then repeat the combination.

tricks of the trade
Nobody looks cool doing these so just get them done and remember that warming up helps improve your performance later on.

kettlebell moves

A few points to remember before beginning these exercises:

- Unless noted otherwise the start position for each move is feet hip width apart, shoulders pulled back and ribs lifted.
- A 'split stance' is an alternative foot position in which one foot is placed forward and the other to the rear, both at hip width apart.
- The grip on the majority of exercises is an 'over-grip' with the thumb and forefinger in the corner of the handle rather than in the centre.
- The 'rack position' is when the kettlebell is held on the back of the forearm.
- 'Bottoms up' refers to when the kettlebell is held upside down.
- Any move that is performed with one hand should always be repeated using the other hand.

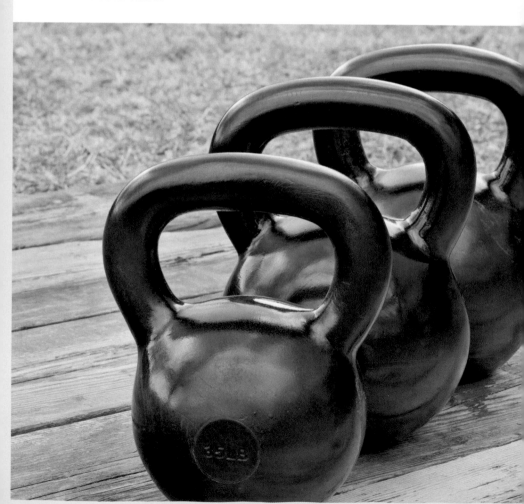

stability

exercise 7 one arm row

● **stability**

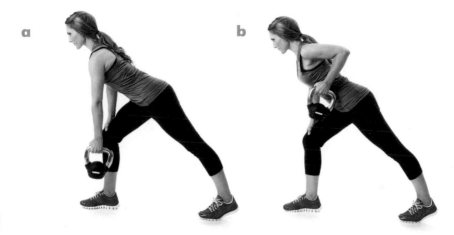

a
b

There is a definite crossover between some dumbbell exercises and what can be achieved using kettlebells. Though we predominately use kettlebells at speed and with a swing, it shouldn't mean we neglect the fact that they are equally challenging when used vertically rather than through an arc. In addition, the reality is that in the 'stability phase' many new users benefit more from static stability to help them become more aware of their body in motion.

● Stand with a split stance and bend forwards from the hips. The kettlebell is next to the front foot.
● Lift the kettlebell up to chest height and lower under control.
● Aim to have movement in the shoulder and upper back rather than just the arm.

> **tricks of the trade**
> You can rest your spare hand on your knee as shown but only lightly. Gripping the leg or pushing with that arm might seem like it's helping you balance but it will turn off some of the beneficial stability demands. For an increased challenge keep the hand off the leg throughout.

exercise 8 front squat

● **stability**

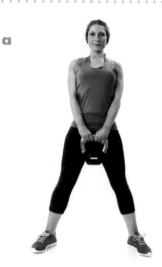

a

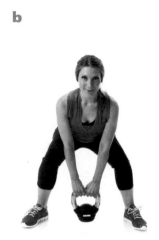

b

Are all squats equal? No, especially when performed holding a kettlebell, as very subtle changes to where and how you hold it will affect the sensation and outcomes of the squat. For example, if you hold the kettlebell away from the body, you will activate more muscle in you back and, by holding it upside down by the horns, the arms and shoulders become more engaged.

● Hold the kettlebell between hip and shoulder height (the higher you hold it the harder the exercise).
● If you opt for hip height as shown in the picture, the kettlebell will almost touch the floor when squatting, but if you opt to hold it at chest height then it stays there through the whole movement.

tricks of the trade

As you squat down, round your shoulders forward and as you stand up squeeze your shoulder blades together – it feels great and is good for your posture.

exercise 9 upright row

● **stability**

a 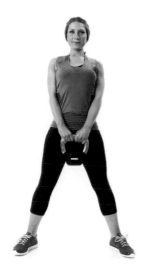 b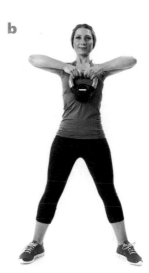

As a rule one arm exercises will be tougher than two so with this move you might find that a lighter kettlebell doesn't feel very challenging. However, this movement pattern is a good one to include in most programmes because it encourages scapular retraction (pulling your shoulders back), which is always a good thing.

● Stand in a regular feet apart position but with the feet turned out slightly.
● Holding the kettlebell with both hands, start with it at the waist, then lift the weight up to chest height.
● In the upper position the elbows are raised higher than the weight. Lower and repeat.

tricks of the trade
Be very critical of this simple move – it's easy to let the elbows creep forwards so aim to keep them out of your eye line.

exercise 10 outside foot pick-up

• stability

a
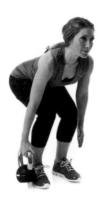

b
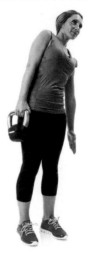

A very wise man once said: 'If you can't explain something simply, then you don't understand it well enough yourself.' Functional training presents so many personal trainers with this exact problem. When I ask personal trainers 'what is functional training?', they often ramble on about 'deep muscle', and 'picking up heavy bags'. However, I simply explain it as skills and movements that relate to how you aim to move in everyday life. Well, here you have the perfect exercise to demonstrate that – actions speak louder than words!

- Holding the kettlebell in one hand, stand with the feet hip width apart.
- Squat down as low as you can – but ensure the depth comes from bending the legs not from a forward bow.
- When you have stood up fully, add a side bend away from the hand with the weight in it.

tricks of the trade

Make sure you squat down low on every repetition – not just the first three when you are thinking about good technique.

exercise 11 straight leg dead lift

● **stability**

a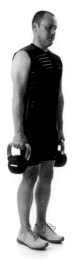

b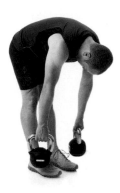

This is an exercise that everyone should do. With every repetition, the hamstrings, glutes and lower back muscles are worked in a way that not only challenges them but also helps protect them from sustaining injury in the future.

- If you have two matching kettlebells, hold one in each hand; if not, do half the reps with the weight in one hand then swap.
- Bend forward from the waist rather than the legs and spine.
- When you reach the limit of your hamstring flexibility, pause for a second then stand up.

tricks of the trade
Controlling your breathing is a key part of this move: breathe out slowly on the way down and in on the way up. Also try and focus on a fixed point as this will help you balance.

exercise 12 hip hinge with kettlebell

● stability

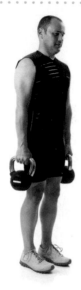

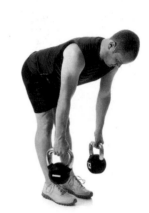

Visually this is similar to the dead lift, however the feet are closer together in this version. Standing with the feet overly wide is an annoying habit you see happening in many gyms, so, to counteract the effects of the wide stance (glute activation rather than inner thigh), the hip hinge should be performed with the feet set close together.

- Start with your feet close together and legs straight.
- Brace the abdominals (this means clench but don't suck in).
- Bend forward from the hips and avoid rounding the shoulders to help you get extra depth as this is counter-productive.

tricks of the trade

Controlling your breathing is a key part of this move because the slow breath out turns your lungs into a solid stabilising unit inside of your torso. Breathe out slowly on the way down and in on the way up.

exercise 13 windmill dead lift

● stability

a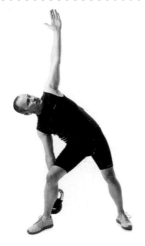

b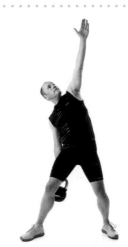

I'm sure that when the phrase 'core training' started to be used in the fitness industry in the late 1990s devotees of kettlebell training must have looked at the techniques and thought 'we have been doing that stuff for years' – it's true. However, in main stream fitness this was really the first time that we started to appreciate the need to move through all three planes of motion.

This move integrates two previous no-nos in that it includes rotation and forward flexion with straight legs.

● Practise this move without a weight first to establish your range of motion.
● Stand with your feet at 90 degrees to each other. If you are holding the kettlebell in your right hand, you need to bend your right leg as you lower the kettlebell towards the floor. Your left leg needs to stay straight (but not locked) as you bend up and down.
● Throughout the up and down phase of the move, keep looking up at the raised arm.

tricks of the trade

Most people are better at this move on one side, so make sure you practise on your 'bad' side without the weight until your range of motion is matched on both sides.

63

exercise 14 one handed floor press (mid section of a Turkish get up)

• **stability**

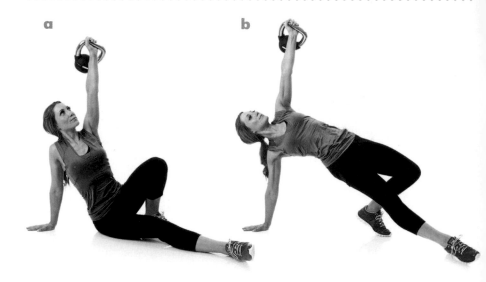

a   b

Not all functional exercises can be directly related back to an everyday movement and this is one of them. By combining bodyweight challenges and the use of external forces (the kettlebell), however, we can create (invent) movements that because of their 'ingredients' work the body efficiently and effectively.

- Sit with one leg bent and the other (top leg) straight.
- Hold the kettlebell in the rack position above you.
- With your bodyweight on the grounded hand and straight leg, lift the torso up as high as you can while keeping the kettlebell still. Lower the hip and repeat.

tricks of the trade
Almost everybody can drive their hips up higher than they think they can, so don't only think about the kettlebell as your body weight is just as important.

exercise 15 single leg side squat, kettlebell at chest

● **stability**

a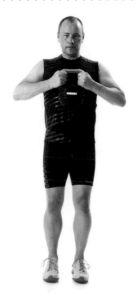

b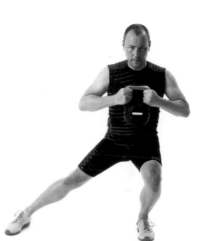

When is one leg better than two? When the goal is all-round core muscle activation rather than lifting the biggest weights. As soon as you stand on one foot, the body throws more nerve stimulation and lateral forces at the working muscles than it does when the load is divided between both feet/legs, making this move an 'A-list celebrity' in the world of leg exercises.

- Holding the kettlebell by the horns and at chest height, stand on one foot.
- Bend the supporting leg and glide the free leg out to the side.
- Focus on keeping the weighted leg in line with your hip and foot.

tricks of the trade

This is the king of 'butt cheek' exercises. Facing a mirror, watch yourself during the move to ensure that the working leg (knee) tracks straight ahead on every repetition.

exercise 16 side bends, arms above head

● **stability**

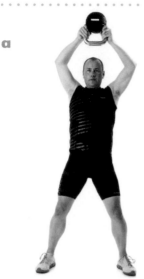

a

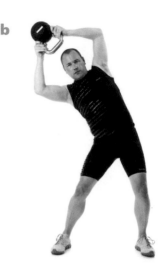

b

In previous books I have included a section on exercises that are a waste of your time. Side bends holding dumbbells was one of those exercises, based on the fact that unless the weights are seriously heavy the move will have very little effect. But it's surprising what a difference moving the load can make, so this version gets the thumbs up.

● Hold the kettlebell by the horns in front of you, then lift it above your head (bottom up).
● Lean to one side keeping your legs straight (the weight will feel heavier as soon as you lean).
● The shoulder muscles should remain static with all the leaning coming from your waist.

tricks of the trade

A word of caution: this move is much harder than side bends with the weight at your waist, so keep the side bend small until you have acclimatised to the effects of holding the weight above your head.

exercise 17 single arm swing

• stability

a

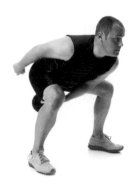

b

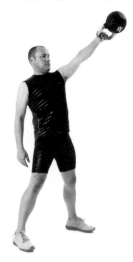

This is the 'classic' kettlebell exercise but not automatically the first one that you should try. Kettlebells need to be treated with respect – because this move includes the demands of both speed and a single handed grip, it's best to attempt this only after you have gotten to grips with the unique characteristics of kettlebells and how they feel when moving both slowly and at speed.

- Begin with the kettlebell hanging in front of you, bend your legs and start the weight swinging (the first swing just gets the weight moving).
- Keep your arm long and hinge at the waist so the kettlebell goes through your legs; at this point, the thumb of your gripping hand should be pointing upwards.
- Now drive the kettlebell forwards and up by using your legs and hips.
- When the kettlebell reaches shoulder height, let it fall back through the legs and repeat.

tricks of the trade

When you get this action right the kettlebell should feel 'weightless' at the top of the move because all the power has came from your legs rather than your shoulder muscles.

exercise 18 two arm swing

● **stability**

a   b

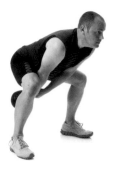
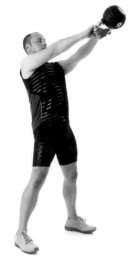

There are some things in life that look easy, but often when you first try them they are harder than they look – riding a bike, rollerblading and swimming are among these skills and so is this classic kettlebell exercise. I often see this move performed badly in gyms so pay close attention to your technique – you will find that when you do get it right, it feels both natural and oddly relaxed.

● Begin with the kettlebell hanging in front of you, bend your legs and start the weight swinging (the first swing just gets the weight moving).
● Keep your arms long and hinge at the waist so the kettlebell goes through your legs.
● Now drive the kettlebell forwards and up by using your legs and hips.
● When the kettlebell reaches shoulder height, control the weight as it falls back through the legs and repeat.

tricks of the trade

If you have got this correct at the top of the swing, the weight should 'relax' giving you time to prepare for the next swing.

strength

exercise 19 swing around the body

● **stability** ● **strength**

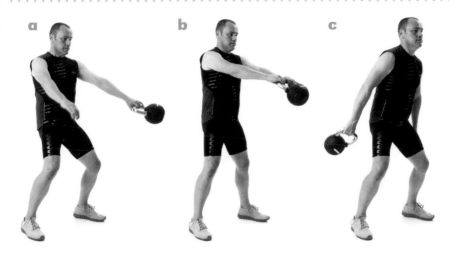

a   b   c

I tell all my trainers that when teaching some exercises the best way is to 'learn it, then work it'. Basically this means getting the technique right before you think about adding any intensity. This move deserves such respect! If you 'miss' when you pass from hand to hand, then that weight is going to go flying so make sure you have plenty of space and that you are on a floor surface that isn't too precious.

● Start with the weight in one hand and your feet shoulder width apart.
● Swing the kettlebell in front of you and swap hands.
● Immediately reach behind you with the spare hand to be ready to receive the weight as you swing it around your body.

tricks of the trade

In this move every muscle between your shoulders and knees is working but the only part you want tensed is your grip – relax everything else and just let the movement flow.

exercise 20 shoulder press

● **stability** ● **strength**

a

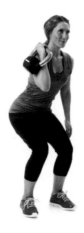

b

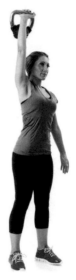

This move is frequently performed with dumbbells or a barbell, however it is harder to do it with a kettlebell of the same weight – why? Simply because the nature of the offset weight in the kettlebell increases the challenge. This is even more the case when you progress to the 'bottom up' version as the kettlebell requires much more stabilisation compared to the dead weight of a dumbbell.

● Bend your legs and lift the weight up to chest height with your elbow bent and the weight close to your body.
● Push the kettlebell straight up until your elbow is almost locked and legs are straight, and pause for a second.
● Lower the weight back down to chest height and repeat.

tricks of the trade

Don't just let the weight be taken over by gravity, lower it back down under control – this doubles the time under tension for the muscles.

exercise 21 overhead squat

• stability • strength

a
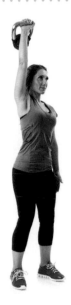

b
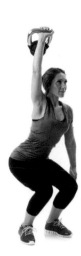

This move is similar to the classic 'prisoner squat', but I don't like the thought of holding the kettlebell behind the head so this is a modified version. It demands all the shoulder and torso stabilising muscle to kick in, but with less risk of banging the back of your head.

- Stand with your feet hip width apart, pick up the kettlebell and hold it in the rack position on a straight arm.
- Squat straight down (avoiding the temptation to lean forwards).
- At the bottom of the squat pause for a second and stand back up.

tricks of the trade

Speed, position and resistance are the three easiest variables for adaptation in any exercise, but varying the position can have the easiest positive effect. This move challenges and improves stability up and down your entire kinetic chain.

exercise 22 swing clean, kettlebell to shoulder

• stability • strength

a   b   c

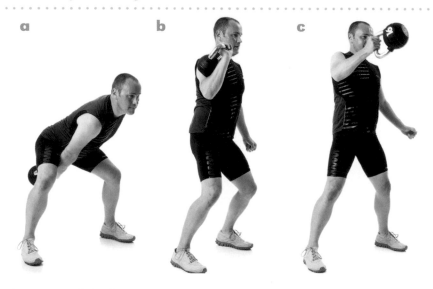

This is one of the first exercises in the portfolio that will make you realise why kettlebells are associated with 'hard core' training.

- 'Release' the weight so it swings through an arc. As it nears its lowest point, bend your knees.
- Drive back up using your hips and legs. As the weight reaches chest height, allow the handle to slide in your hand so the ball of the kettlebell swings over the hand and comes to a rest on the back of your forearm.
- Hold the weight close to your body in this rack position.
- Punch the weight away from you to start the swing action again and repeat.

tricks of the trade

Going from the rack to the swing position will probably seem rather 'drastic' the first few times you try it but as you learn to control the kettlebell you will quickly master the skill of how and when to decelerate the kettlebell.

exercise 23 military press

● **stability** ● **strength**

a
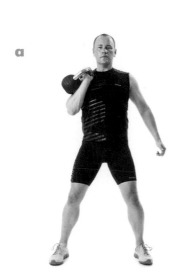

b
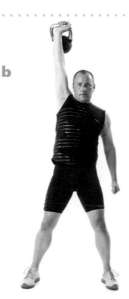

Whether you perform this move with either one or two kettlebells, it is one of the most satisfying exercises I know probably because the 'push' phase is short and sharp, and when you get the kettlebell to the highest position, you can feel the entire body contributing to the action. Unlike a regular shoulder press, the military version doesn't have any drive coming from the legs, instead the legs just stabilise the body.

● Clean the weight to shoulder height and hold in the rack position.
● Keep a straight (imaginary) line through the centre of your body.
● Push the weight up so that it stays in line with your shoulder (rather than above your head).
● Lower the weight under control and repeat.

tricks of the trade

If you are using anything less than your heaviest kettlebell, then this move needs to be performed quickly with a short sharp puff of expired air coming out of your mouth when you get to the top position.

exercise 24 swing into pull at top

• stability • strength

a   b   c

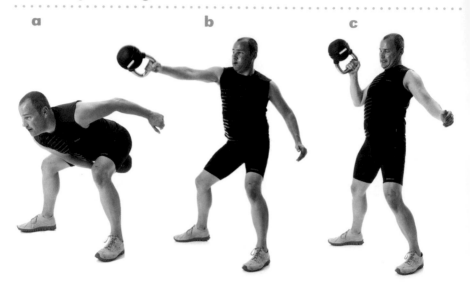

This is a fantastic move – not only does it make you work through multiple planes of motion, it also has the deviation from the arc when you pull the kettlebell towards you. It's another of those moves that doesn't instantly relate to anything you do in your everyday life, but in terms of conditioning the body for any eventuality, it rocks!

- Practise this move first without the weight as it is important the pull happens at chest height rather than head height.
- Swing the weight through your legs and up to chest height.
- At the top of the arc, pull the weight towards your body keeping the bottom of the weight at 90 degrees to the floor, then push the weight back quickly so that it can drop down through the arc again.

tricks of the trade

The pull section of this move is easy so don't use too much force – save it for pushing the weight back out into its arc.

exercise 25 single arm windmill

● **stability** ● **strength**

a
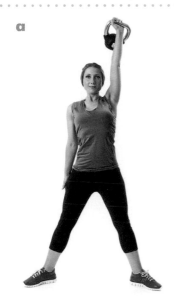

b
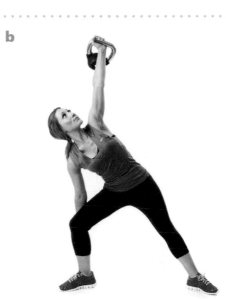

Though the supporting leg on this exercise is bent which reduces the flexibility required, this move is still a fantastic exercise for activating the 'team' of muscles that stabilise the lower back and pelvis.

● Hold the weight with a straight arm (left hand) in the rack position above your head.
● Bend the right leg and reach down the side of your left inner thigh, aiming to reach the floor.
● To stand up again, initiate the movement with a quick push from the right leg then let the torso take over and stand up smoothly.

tricks of the trade

There are some exercises where holding your breath is advantageous but with this move a slow exhalation on the way down is better simply because when the breath is held the lungs form a solid 'mass' which would restrict your ability to bend down and flex through the torso.

exercise 26 hammer curl (bicep curl bottom up)

• stability • strength

a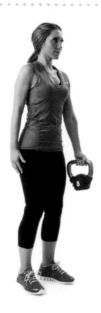

b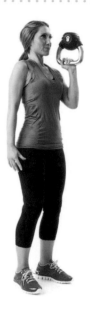

This move almost fits in to the 'hard for the sake of it' section but it manages to be challenging without damaging – and it does fabulous things to your grip strength (which in turn helps you with every other lift you do).

- Stand holding the kettlebell hanging at your side.
- Aim to keep your elbow close to the side of your body, then curl the weight up using your bicep muscle.
- When the elbow joint is fully flexed, slowly reverse the movement.

tricks of the trade

A word of warning: don't expect to be able to lift as much as you can when doing a regular dumbbell bicep curl, but revel in the fact you are doing great things for your grip strength.

exercise 27 clean and press

• stability • strength

a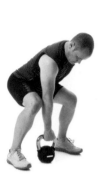

b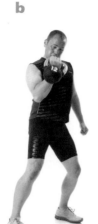

c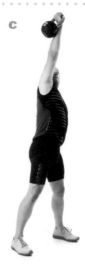

When I spend time with trainee personal trainers I often feel they don't really understand what they are talking about because they are struggling with the new vocabulary that they think they need to use – instead of saying 'bend' and 'twist', they start talking about 'sagittal planes' and 'frontal planes', etc. Maybe they feel this impresses people; frankly, I think it puts people off.

On this move, let's keep it simple as you have done it a thousand times before – squat, bend and push.

● Place the weight between your feet and squat down.
● Grasp the weight in the corner of the handle, then pull it swiftly upwards.
● When the weight reaches chest height, transfer to the rack position and without losing momentum push the weight up to its highest position then reverse the action.

tricks of the trade

Think about the weight going up and down in a straight vertical line. The aim here is not to 'punctuate' the movement but rather turn it into one smooth action – you don't have to touch the weight to the floor between each repetition.

exercise 28 single leg dead lift, kettlebell to foot

• stability • strength

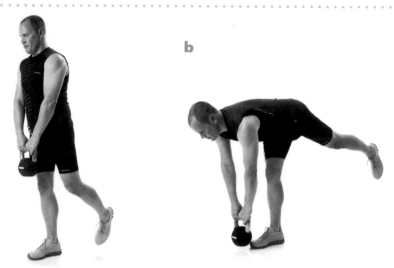

A good friend of mine carries out research at a top American university specialising in finding the simplest way of achieving results. After extensive analysis, this move became one of the top five 'must do' exercises for back care, strength and conditioning. However, it's still one of those moves you don't often see being done in the gym (maybe because it takes practice to do it well). Personally, I do this every day; it takes minutes and keeps my back strong and mobile.

- Hold the kettlebell by the horns with both hands.
- Bend forward (hinge) at the waist whilst also lifting one leg up. The kettlebell lowers towards the floor as you bend.
- The perfect technique is to have the lifted leg as high as your head and shoulders when you are bending forwards.

tricks of the trade

Balance can be the biggest challenge during this move. A great trick is to press your tongue against the roof of your mouth as you hinge forward and amazingly your balance will improve (due to muscles in your neck and shoulders being activated).

exercise 29 hefo reach with kettlebell

• stability • strength

a
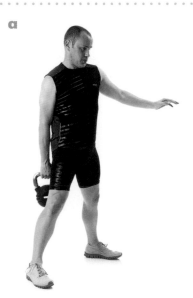

b
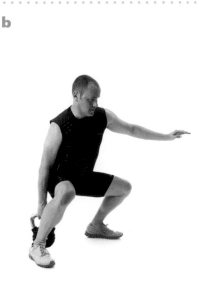

There are plenty of exercises that you can do with both dumbbells and kettlebells, however this is a great example of one that feels 'right' when you do it with a kettlebell rather than a dumbbell.

- Stand with your feet apart in a wide stance (plie position).
- Hang the weight behind you in one hand, squat down with both legs and lean at the waist towards the side on which you are holding the weight.
- Stand up by driving up with your glutes, inner thighs and hamstrings.

tricks of the trade

This exercise is one of the moves I feel can help protect you from injury because it takes you through a movement pattern that doesn't feature in many other exercises yet is fantastic for 'teaching' the body to cope with extension, torsion and recoil – which in my opinion makes it fantastic!

exercise 30 pendulum swing 6–3 & 6–9

● stability ● strength

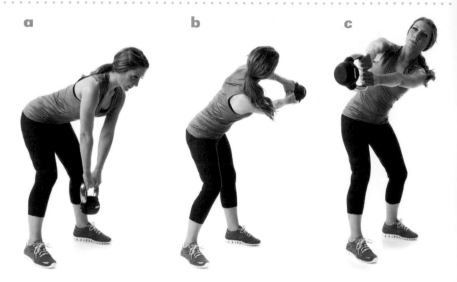

a   b   c

One of my biggest frustrations with personal trainers and instructors is that they 'over coach' exercises by telling their client how to move. Every client looks and moves differently and I often think the personal trainers are simply trying to look busy – if it feels 'good', then you are probably doing it right.

● Stand with your feet slightly wider than hip width apart with the kettlebell between your feet (6 o'clock position).
● Bend down (hip hinge) and hold the weight keeping your arms straight.
● The drive (force) to lift the weight up to the 3 o'clock position comes from rotating briskly with your torso.
● Try to lower the weight with some control stopping at the bottom before repeating on the other side.

tricks of the trade

This move has 'individualism' written all over it because everybody looks slightly different when they do it – so fear not if your feet twist or you don't lift it as high as in the picture. 'If you are moving, you are improving'.

exercise 31 single leg squat, kettlebell bottom up

• **stability** • **strength**

a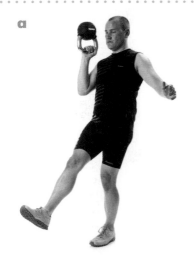

b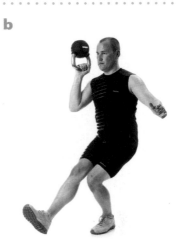

The single leg squat part of this move is a fantastic way of improving your squats if you are currently quad dominant (which means you don't activate your glute max and hamstrings enough when you squat), and the 'bottom up' part of the move fires up the muscles above your pelvis and up through the spine.

- Perfect the single leg squat before adding the kettlebell, then progress to holding the weight on the same side as the leg you are working (holding it in the opposite hand is more challenging).
- With the kettlebell bottom up, keep it at chest height then bend the working leg.
- Squat down only as far as you can maintain good posture, then drive back up focusing on using your glutes and hamstrings.

tricks of the trade

This is another of those moves that deserves the title of 'super move' as it incorporates so many good ingredients into one exercise. So, if you are busy, save all the clever stuff for when you have more time and do a few sets of this fantastic exercise!

exercise 32 push press with half squat

• stability • strength

a

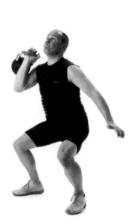

b

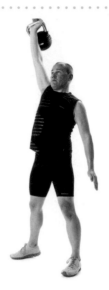

Any one sided exercise is going to create contralateral forces (a force that crosses over the body's imaginary centre line) rather than just directing force symmetrically (or if you want the technical jargon, ipso-laterally). Done either one or two handed, this is a very raw movement which conditions the entire body.

As this exercise includes a drive phase from the legs, it is preferable to use a heavier weight than you would for regular shoulder presses.

- Hold the kettlebell in the rack position with your knees bent.
- Now drive the weight (or weights) straight up.
- Look up and as you reach the top of the movement with the weight simultaneously push up onto your toes. Lower the weight and repeat.

tricks of the trade

If you have two kettlebells of the same weight, you can do this as a double handed exercise, but doing it one side at a time can actually have additional benefits if you define intensity as 'stability plus strength required' rather than just basing it on how much weight you are lifting.

exercise 33 single leg hip hinge, kettlebell to foot

● **stability** ● **strength**

a

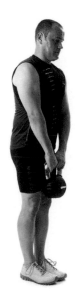

b

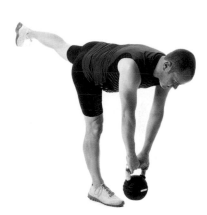

While at first glance this move looks similar to the single leg dead lift (exercise 28), it feels completely different simply because the weight is moving against its instinctive route (straight down with gravity).

● Hold the kettlebell by the horns with an over-grip.
● Extend your left leg behind you, bending forward at the waist as the foot leaves the ground.
● The weight should now move towards the floor but stay closely in line with your body as it lowers. Keep moving until you reach your maximum range of motion then reverse the action.
● Ultimately the working leg will stay straight while the unloaded leg and torso will be parallel to the ground.

> ### tricks of the trade
>
> All the hip hinge moves were introduced to me by people who practised yoga in the late 1990s. Before that I'd avoided anything that required forward flexion and straight legs as I was under the impression it was 'contra-indicated'. In the fitness industry attitudes often change in regard to information we may have previously considered correct – it doesn't mean that we were wrong back then, just that we now have a better understanding of how the body works. So my advice is: don't dismiss it until you have tried it. Old habits die hard so don't be surprised if people ask you if this is safe, it is.

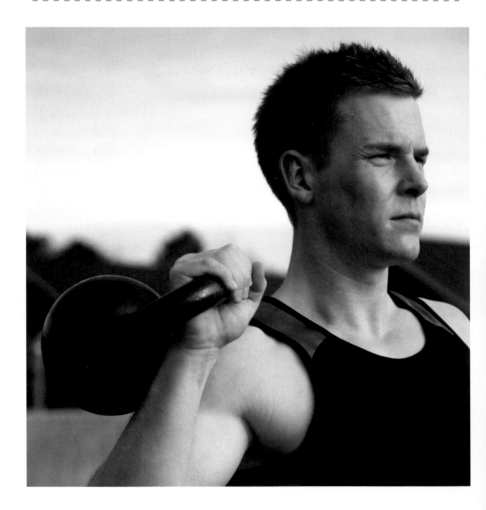

exercise 34 halo, circling kettlebell around head

• stability • strength

a

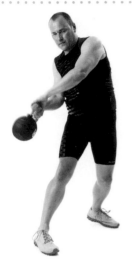

b

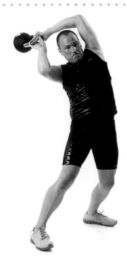

The emphasis here is actually to move the kettlebell around your shoulders, rather than just around your head. This of course means that mobility in the shoulders is essential but the good news is that doing this move will also help loosen up tight shoulders as well as give you strength gains.

- Hold the kettlebell by the horns but with your palms facing forwards.
- The emphasis is on 'rolling' your arms around your head and shoulders rather than lifting the kettlebell up high.
- Try to generate movement in the whole of your torso rather than just moving your arms.
- Do all the repetitions in one direction before going the other way; that way you can build up some beneficial momentum.

tricks of the trade

This move is great but you really must follow my advice and 'learn it, then work it': rather than starting straight away with a kettlebell, first practise the technique with something more forgiving like a rolled up towel or soft ball – that way if you get it wrong, you'll still be smiling.

exercise 35 sots press

• stability • strength

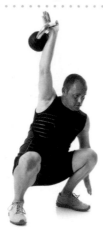

a

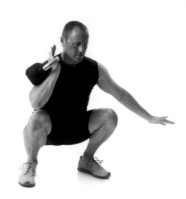

b

As I've said before, no exercises make it in to this book simply because they are hard; everything has to be simple, achievable and functional – this move is all three.

Legend has it that the inventor of this move had reached the stage where none of his kettlebells were heavy enough anymore, so he looked for new ways to add challenges to his lifts (pushes). The deep squat position certainly achieves that but at the same time it cleverly introduces a whole level of functionality to strength training because when you think about it not every movement in real life starts from a standing position.

- Lift the kettlebell above you and hold in the rack position. Squat down deep with your feet shoulder width apart.
- Lean away from the weighted side and press the weight above you.
- Lower the weight while simultaneously moving your torso back towards the centre of the squat then repeat.

tricks of the trade

This squat is the deepest you will ever do so be prepared to 'bail out' by putting the weight on the floor while you are still squatting rather than when you have stood back up.

exercise 36 frontal swing, kettlebell between split stance legs

• stability • strength

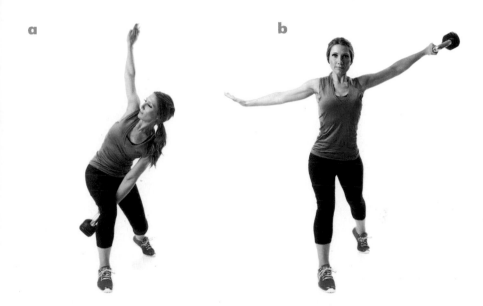

The entire nature of exercising with a kettlebell means you are trying to accelerate it and then control the deceleration. The most common exercises all move vertically or through an arc in front of you – this little creation, however, swings at you from the side and demands you stabilise with the less dominant adductor and abductor muscles in the legs and generate the force with the muscle in your waist rather than your glutes.

- Step forward with your right leg into a lunge while holding the kettlebell in your left hand.
- With the weight hanging down in line with your torso, swing the weight through your legs and then out to the side (the first 2 or 3 reps are used to generate momentum).
- The weight will want to swing through an arc so you need to direct it through your legs then power it up to shoulder height. Remember this is powered by the legs and torso not the arms.

> **tricks of the trade**
>
> There's no easy way of learning this move but the best way I have found is to do it without the weight first and to go through the move in very slow motion – you might feel silly if you are in the gym, but it's worth it.

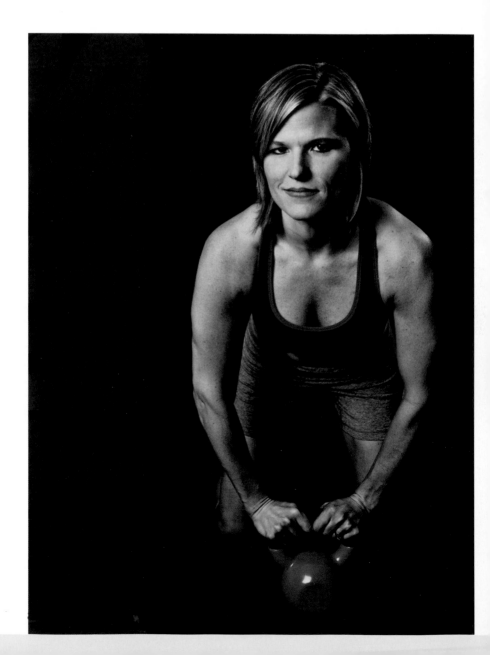

power

exercise 37 dead lift clean

● **stability** ● **strength** ● **power**

a
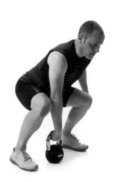

b
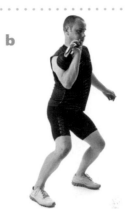

Dead lift means 'straight up' so the weight does not swing, it moves vertically. This is easier with a dumbbell because, with a kettlebell, you have to spin it around on its own axis. If you learn it in 'real time' rather than trying to slow it down, this tends to make the move a bit easier.

● The first repetition starts from the floor, but from then on, lower the weight close to the ground but without touching the floor.
● Drive upwards using the legs, creating enough momentum to get the weight to chest height and flip it over into the rack position.
● Pause and remember that on the way down you need to decelerate the weight to avoid hitting the floor.

tricks of the trade

As we start to explore the power generating moves, I hope that you have resisted the temptation to skip the previous exercises and go straight on the 'harder' moves – if you have, you will have missed out on the opportunity for your body to establish 'muscle memory' which is the subconscious development of movement skills. It's human nature to think that the 'tough stuff' will be more beneficial, but when it comes to the body it really is all about quality over quantity, so 'earn it, then work it'.

exercise 38 swing snatch, kettlebell above head

• stability • strength • power

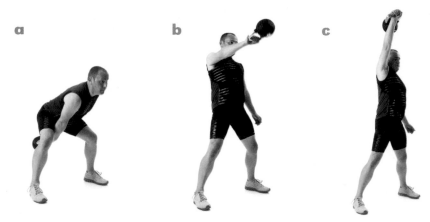

a   b   c

This move is fantastically functional if you break it down to its individual components – if you think in terms of 'transferable skills' rather than mimicking every day movements, functional exercise is so much easier to understand.

By this stage you know how to swing but adding the snatch means you are dealing with the deceleration of the weight when it is above you rather than out in front so this increases the challenge enormously.

- In preparation, swing the weight to chest height for 3 to 4 reps.
- The snatch happens when the weight is above you so as the weight reaches head height slide your hand under the weight so that it transfers on to the back of your forearm.
- At the highest point you need to rapidly decelerate, then swing back down to reverse the arc.

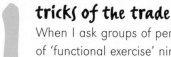

tricks of the trade

When I ask groups of personal trainers to give me their interpretation of 'functional exercise' nine times out of ten they will talk about doing movements that look similar to everyday tasks like picking up bags, etc. However, they are missing the point. This move is fantastically functional even though it doesn't resemble moves that occur in the average person's day.

exercise 39 plunges holding by the horns

• stability • strength

a

b

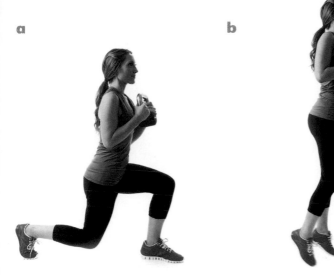

When is a lunge not a lunge? When it's a plunge! A fast-moving kettlebell is normally swung through an arc to create power in your torso but performing these plunges while gripping the horns of the kettlebell can invoke powerful contractions from every muscle involved.

- Step into a front lunge while holding the kettlebell in front of you (the weight should be slightly towards the side of the back leg).
- Jump upwards while simultaneously lifting the weight just a little.
- As you swap legs move the weight across the centre line of your body and as you land decelerate then repeat.

tricks of the trade

I often see this move performed with a lack of energy – if both feet don't leave the ground with a jump then it's a lunge and not a plunge. The trick is to focus on jumping as high as you can and then rather than landing rigid, land softly so that your knee sinks really close to the ground before you do another explosive jump up for the next repetition.

exercise 40 one-handed cross chop

• stability • strength • power

a

b

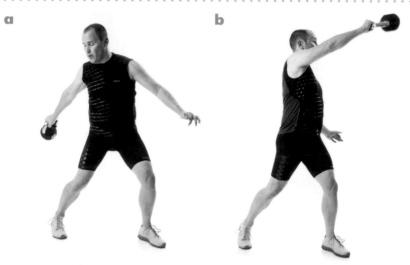

This is a personal trainer '101' exercise as it is always the example used to explain the three different planes of motion that the body moves through (sagittal, frontal and transverse) as it incorporates all three. However, the demo is normally done using a medicine ball. This version is a massive step up in terms of the intensity and body control (skill) that is required to perform it well.

- Stand in a lunge position with the left foot forward. Hold the weight in your right hand (only do this move with the weight in the outside hand or you will hit your leg).
- Brace the shoulders and rotate quickly towards the front leg and lift the weight up to chest height.
- As you reach the highest position, reverse the rotation and recoil in the other direction. Make sure the weight is held high enough so that it doesn't hit your back leg.

tricks of the trade

This move is enhanced even more if you follow the kettlebell with your eyes as it goes through its arc.

exercise 41 the Andrea

● stability ● strength ● power

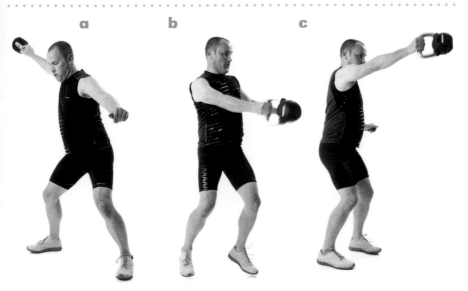

a b c

I'm sure this move has a technical name but with hundreds of moves in my head sometimes I find it easier to remember things by word association. This exercise was taught to me by a fantastic Brazilian athlete I work with called Andrea so what better name to give it!

When you start to learn it the foot movement resembles a skip (two foot to one foot jump), but when you master it you can jump both feet at the same time.

● Practice this entire move without the kettlebell first, then add the weight when you have mastered the co-ordination.
● Stand with your feet apart and with the weight in your right hand. Swing the kettlebell laterally to head height then let your right arm swing down across the front of your body. As the weight swings across your body, you then jump (picture b) so that your body turns 90 degrees in the air and you land with your feet in a new position (picture c).
● The kettlebell will continue to swing until it reaches head height, you then let it drop back towards the side of you body at which point you jump again so that your body and feet return to the position shown in picture a.

tricks of the trade

The jumping part of this move (called 'firing') is fantastic for developing dynamic strength so work on it as an individual exercise by jumping 180 degrees rather than just 90 degrees.

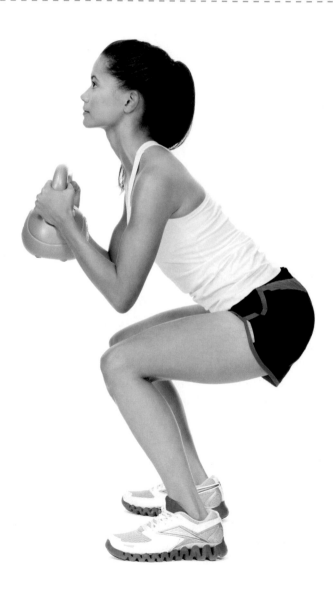

exercise 42 clean and step back

• **stability** • **strength** • **power**

a
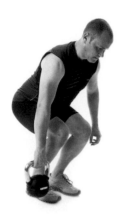

b
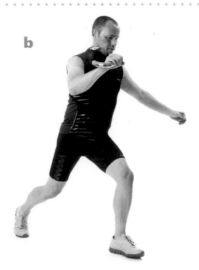

This is an excellent move which has the ability to be performed in a number of different ways by making subtle changes. You can do it with the opposite leg to arm or the same arm to leg, as well as by shifting your bodyweight more or less onto the front or back foot. Some moves are more subtle than others and this is one of them.

- Stand with your feet close together and the kettlebell placed next to the front foot.
- Quickly lift the weight up straight into the racked position and simultaneously step back with the right foot.
- As you lower the weight, step the foot forwards again.

tricks of the trade

In terms of being functional I think it scores top marks in particular because of the foot movements. In real life we move our feet when we are lifting objects, it's only in the gym we seem to create 'rules' to limit this. Personal trainers would do well to remember this – clients get bored of being told off all the time.

exercise 43 coronal arc (hammer twist)

• stability • strength • power

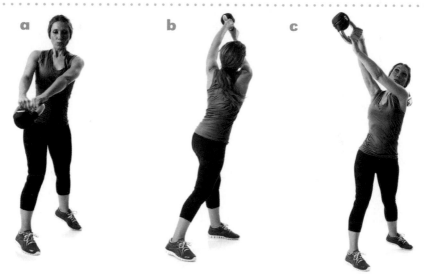

'Coronal' is an alternative name for the frontal plane of motion and for me is a more logical term as it's easy to misinterpret 'frontal' as meaning in front whereas in fact it refers to the imaginary line through the middle of the body. With this move it's best to start with a lighter weight than you would assume you should use because, when your arms are extended above your head while you are bending sideways, it will feel heavier than you expect.

- Holding the kettlebell by the horns, twist your upper body so the weight is outside of your hip.
- Keeping the arms long and straight, lift the weight outwards then over your head; the kettlebell should travel through a large arc above you.
- Decelerate the weight as it reaches the opposite hip and repeat the action.

tricks of the trade

You simply cannot do this move gently. Go as fast as you can whilst maintaining control of the weight.

exercise 44 the jerk

● **stability** ● **strength** ● **power**

a   b   c

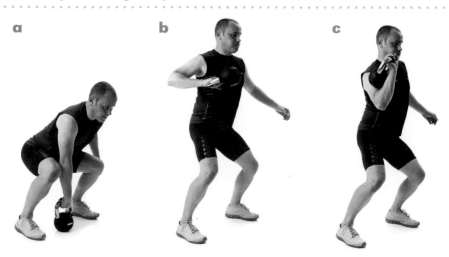

This move is best performed using a matching pair of kettlebells but I understand that many people training at home will only have one of each weight. However, this got me thinking: 'Is it a problem to push with different size weights in each hand?' The answer is 'no'. Just because you don't see it happening in gyms doesn't mean it is wrong (far from it). In fact if you think about it, the gym is probably the only time you push anything with both hands and get identical resistance on each side. The only caveat with this move, therefore, is that you must always swap sides so that you even things up.

● The aim is to quickly lift the weight up to chest/shoulder height in one swift movement using power from your legs. From the start position, pull the weight up vertically.
● As it begins to run out of momentum (picture b) you need to dip down with your legs very quickly so that you control the weight (this quick squatting action is called the 'catch'), you then simultaneously flip the kettlebell to the rack position (picture c).
● Once in the rack position, you pause for a moment then flip the kettlebell off the back of the forearm and lower the weight back towards the floor for the next repetition.

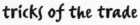

tricks of the trade

All the moves that involve a catch are helpful for teaching the body to protect our spine – catching the weight with your legs rather than taking your back muscles by surprise is always going to be preferable.

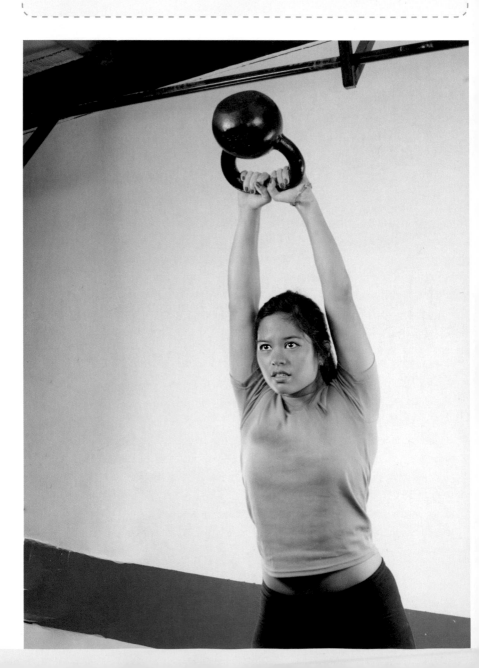

exercise 45 skater swing

● **stability** ● **strength**

a   b

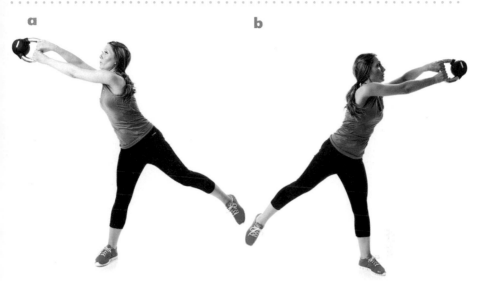

Here's a great example of what happens when you bother to spend time thinking about exercises rather than just doing the same old 'stuff' over and over again. The swing element of the move is relatively standard with the force coming from the recoil you get after creating torsion in your torso. The lifting of the foot increases the 'fun' element and, as with any exercise, as soon as you add balance the effects increase.

● Stand with your feet just over shoulder width apart and the kettlebell held by the horns in front of you.
● Shift (glide) your body weight side to side and start to let the weight swing.
● The weight shouldn't lift any higher than your ribs – the main objective is to be smooth and controlled rather than fast and furious.

tricks of the trade

Skaters have the most superb balance and core strength so this flowing movement should be included even if you don't really 'feel it' – not everything is supposed to be hard!

exercise 46 cross chop catch, step forward

● **stability** ● **strength** ● **power**

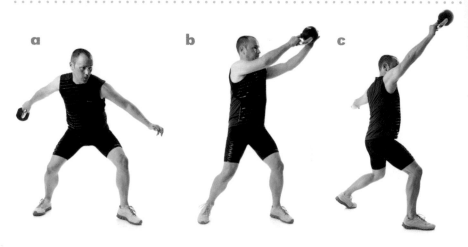

The 'step forward' part of this move is a small step rather than a lunge. As with all kettlebell swings, the 'lift' comes from the legs and torso rather than the arms so the aim here is to drive forward with the back leg, then literally put the brakes on with the opposite hand and the front leg.

● This move is similar to the one-handed cross chop (exercise 40), but it is performed faster and you take a very quick step forward and back at the top of the movement.
● Stand with your feet apart holding the kettlebell in your right hand and at your side. Build up some momentum with some preparatory swings from side to side across the front of your body. Increase the speed of the swing then at the top of the movement, 'catch' the weight (picture b) with your left hand to slow it down.
● While the kettlebell is at its highest point (picture c), make a very quick step forward (with your right foot) then as the weight drops down, step quickly back to the start position.

tricks of the trade

Most people instinctively keep the working arm bent to start with – that's fine as the bigger the arc the harder this move becomes so they are effectively learning it before they work it.

exercise 47 one handed swing, release and catch

• stability • strength • power

a
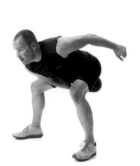

b
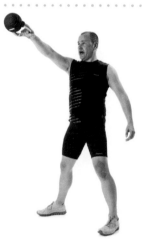

You will know by now that I don't like any exercises that I class as 'circus acts' or juggling simply because the chances of them going wrong outweigh the benefits. But, I like this move because the release and catch phase actually serves a purpose – when you catch the kettlebell, you have to use your energy to control its energy and to me that's classed as exercise rather than just showing off.

- In the swing section of this move, you drive with your legs and hips to power the weight up and through its arc.
- With the weight at shoulder height, lean back slightly pulling the weight towards you and release your grip.
- Keep watching the kettlebell and catch it again; the weight will be higher than when you let go.
- As you catch the weight, you need to absorb the energy and steer the weight back down for the next swing.

tricks of the trade

If catching things in general is a problem for you, catching a kettlebell certainly will be, so I like to practise the release and catch with a tennis ball before contemplating doing it with a weight.

exercise 48 squat snatch

• **stability** • **strength** • **power**

a

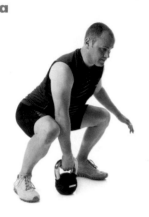

b

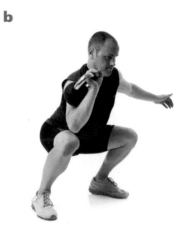

Ideally rehearse this move without the weight as you need to experience the sensation of standing up at speed before you add the weight. The kettlebell you select then needs to be heavy enough to slow you down as you drive up.

This exercise relates very well to the sots press (exercise 35).

- Start with the weight near the floor, swing it through your legs then upwards in an arc.
- Snatch the weight over your hand by driving up hard with your legs, however, rather than standing up, drop back down and squat under the weight, looking up at the weight.
- Stand up fully, then 'un-rack' the kettlebell and roll it back down the front of your body ready for the next repetition.

tricks of the trade

To learn the correct position for the squat section, stand with your back to a wall, slide down it then lift one arm above you – the base of your spine, shoulders and hand should all be touching the wall.

exercise 49 one handed swing and switch hands

• **stability** • **strength** • **power**

a
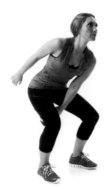

b
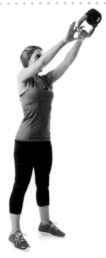

We do this move not because it is clever (which it is) but because switching the weight (force) from one side to the other is a fantastic way of improving core strength as the very best way of improving stability is to make all the muscle around the lumbo pelvic area react to directional changes of force.

- In the swing section of this move, drive up with your legs and hips to power the weight up and through its arc.
- With the weight at shoulder height, lean back slightly pulling the weight towards you and release your grip.
- Keep watching the kettlebell as the weight will be higher than when you released it and catch it again with your other hand. As you catch the weight you need to absorb the energy and steer the weight back down for the next swing.

tricks of the trade

I cannot emphasis enough how important it is to do this move on a floor that you don't mind a kettlebell being dropped on – even the best people miss sometimes.

exercise 50 bottom up snatch

• stability • strength • power

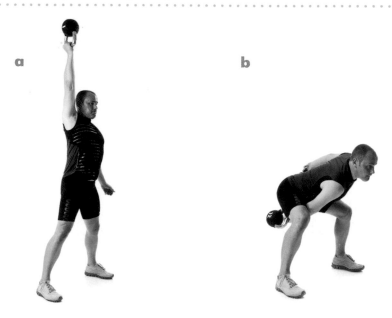

a

b

Most kettlebell moves flow from one repetition straight into the next one but this move benefits from a pause between each rep. The first phase – the snatch – is pretty standard, but when you reach shoulder height and you have started to flip the kettlebell, your shoulder and upper back then have to engage very quickly to balance the weight. Unlike a regular snatch where you let the weight come to a rest on the back of your forearm, you pause with the bottom of the weight pointing straight up to the ceiling.

- With the bottom up moves there is no opportunity to 'relax' at the top of the movement as you have to concentrate to balance the weight.
- Stand feet hip width apart and perform a regular single arm swing, near the top of the swing, twist the kettlebell so that you thumb is pointing behind you.
- With the weight at head height, you now force the weight to change direction towards you and drive it above your head. The handle is now under the weight section. At the top allow the weight to swing back down through its original arc and then repeat.

tricks of the trade

Practise having the weight in the bottom up position and walking and stepping side to side so that you get used to the sensation of the weight getting away from you so that you learn how to correct it.

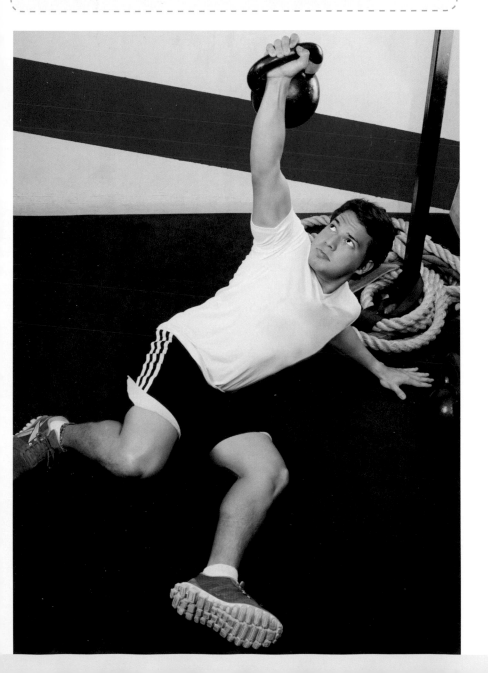

exercise 51 split jerk

• **stability** • **strength** • **power**

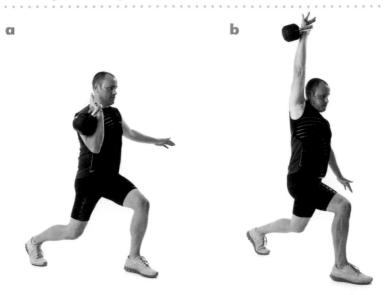

a   b

I think this is a fantastic move because it starts from such an 'off balanced' position. It's a move where it would be easy to over analyse what's working but think of the movement as a whole rather than as a series of individual muscle contractions. If you keep your feet in line rather than split them, the balance challenge increases enormously.

- Stand in a split stance (right leg back) and with the kettlebell in the rack position (using your right hand).
- Drive the weight above your head and simultaneously jump into a split stance landing with the right foot in the forward position.
- Walk the feet back to the start position and repeat the move.

tricks of the trade

When learning Olympic lifting techniques there is a reason we do it with a plastic pipe rather than with a proper bar – because nobody gets this right first time. If you are going to make a beginner's mistake, it's best to do it without a weight in your hand – we are all only human.

exercise 52 pendulum swing non-stop

• stability • strength • power

a   b   c

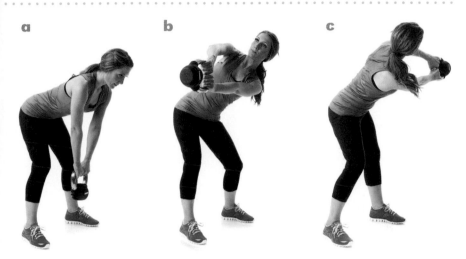

A pendulum swings freely, however, when a kettlebell is involved we need to be in control. Being in the hip hinge position, the legs are not the driving force here; more so the torso is driving and controlling the swinging action. Practise the movement without the weight – i.e. "learn it, then work it".

- Stand with feet slightly wider than hip distance apart with the kettlebell between your feet (6 o'clock position).
- Bend down (hip hinge) and lift the weight off the floor keeping your back flat and arms straight.
- Then using your torso muscles, lift the weight up to the right (9 o'clock position) then quickly drive it back towards the floor and without stopping, swing it up to your left (3 o'clock position). Repeat so the weight continues to swing side to side.

tricks of the trade

There is a real temptation to hold your breath when you do this. Years ago we would have said that was 'bad' for you, but now we understand core stabilisation better we know that it's an instinctive reaction that aides stabilisation – just don't hold it for any longer than one repetition.

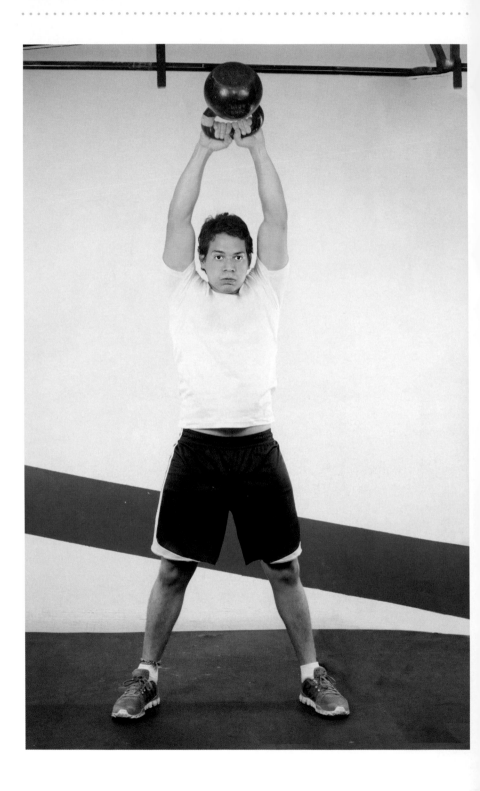

moves to avoid

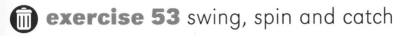

🗑 **exercise 53** swing, spin and catch

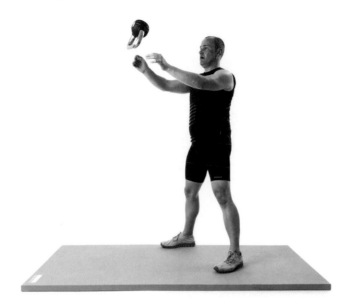

I'm not saying this move doesn't require skill but I think the physical benefits of spinning the kettlebell are negligible. Also, if you don't catch the kettlebell correctly, then there is a real risk of injury to your feet (not to mention damage to flooring).

---

tricks of the trade

Do the one arm swing and switch hands (exercise 49, page 103) instead.

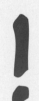 **exercise 54** 'shot putt' press

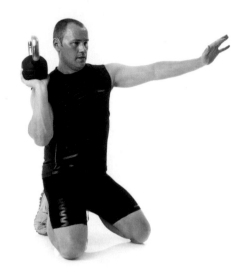

Kettlebell fanatics are a loyal bunch so again I'm sure that there may be some justification for this exercise but realistically you can achieve similar effects (balance and shoulder stability) doing other moves without the risk of dropping the kettlebell – there is a reason for having a handle on a kettlebell, so use it!

> ## **tricks of the trade**
> Do the sots press (exercise 35, page 86) instead.

🗑 exercise 55 throw

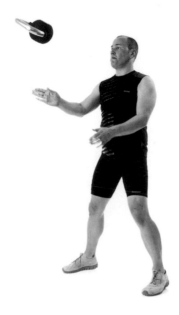

The only people for whom I can justify throws are athletic competitors in the shot, discus or hammer disciplines because it does have physical benefits at their level but also they can do the moves in a proper throwing cage.

> **!** **tricks of the trade**
> Do the coronal arc (or hammer twist, exercise 43, page 96).

exercise 56 extended sit up, sitting on feet and leaning back

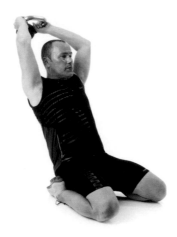

If I ask people why they do this move, the response is generally 'I can really feel it working'. Fine, but is that 'feeling' good or bad? – I've tried this move with no weights, medicine balls and kettlebells and the feeling I get is certainly muscle recruitment in the abdominals but also an unnerving sensation around the knee joint that feels like the patello femoral joint and patella tendon are being put under inappropriate pressure, so for me it's not worth the risk.

 tricks of the trade
Do side bends with arms above ahead (exercise 16, page 66) instead.

exercise 57 any exercise where the kettlebell is balanced on the foot

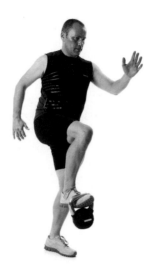

The most innocent exercise of this type I've seen are dips and pull ups with a kettlebell hanging from the foot; the worst is a kettlebell hanging from the foot when the person was in a handstand position trying to do inverted press ups! It might be hard but it's also reckless – only use equipment in the manner it was designed for. There's a reason it's called a handle!

 **tricks of the trade**
Do the Andrea (exercise 41, page 93) instead.

exercise 58 Turkish get up

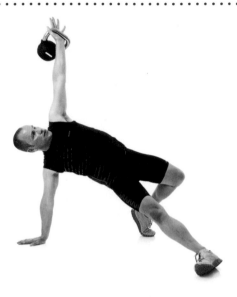

Don't get me wrong, this is a fantastic exercise and I know this is one of the classic kettlebell exercises that personal trainers want to learn as a rite of passage but if you break down the individual components, they all exist in other moves in this book.

So, unless you are a wrestler or MMA fighter then chances are the benefits of a one handed floor to ceiling lift are outweighed by the amount of time it takes to learn. Disagree? Well, the thing is the individual components are easy, it's the stringing of them all together that confuses people. Even without a weight in their hand people struggle to remember the sequence, which is: Lie flat, lift weight, hand out, bend leg, press up to seated position, reposition leg, push up onto one knee, stand up – repeat in the reverse order. See what I mean!

> **tricks of the trade**
> Instead, if you do everything else in this book, you will actually move through the same movement patterns just faster and with a more natural flow.

exercise 59 any move that is 'hard' just for the sake of it

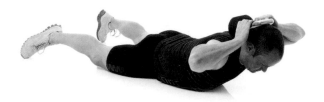

There is a difference between hard work and an exercise that is just 'hard' for the sake of it. It's too easy to get creative with kettlebells and think because you can 'feel it' that it must be good for you. Sadly, often the pain that you feel is the ligaments and tendons straining rather anything productive – so avoid anything that you don't understand or can't justify as being safe and effective.

 tricks of the trade

Again, every move in the rest of this book is simple because it has earned its place and is safe, effective and functional. So do any of the other moves in this book!

3 training with kettlebells

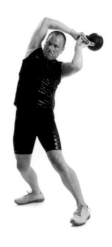

how to use the kettlebell training sessions

· ·

As people become more experienced in training with kettlebells there is a temptation to forego a formal training plan and work through a session training body parts randomly. This can be effective, but human nature dictates that, given the opportunity, we often end up focusing on the parts we like to work rather than the parts we need to work.

The training sessions in this section follow the S.A.F.E. philosophy of progression and are divided into the three basic facets of this system: stability, strength and power. They are sequenced in such a way that if you were an absolute beginner when you started, you should have at least 18 months of progressive exercise experience before you perform the hardest session. So, a novice would first attempt the 15 minute stability session, followed when ready by the 20 minute and then 30 minute sessions. This process could take three to six months. When the stability sessions have been mastered and no longer present a significant challenge, the 15 minute strength session can be attempted, followed when ready by the 20 and 30 minute sessions; again, this process could take three to six months. Having developed stability and strength over this length of time the body will be well-prepared to progress to the power sessions, which follow the same logical progressions. Note: the timings are approximate and include a short warm-up and stretching at the end of the session.

The reality is, of course, that many people are not complete beginners, so Table 2 gives you an idea of where to start depending upon your experience and physical ability.

Table 2 Assessing which training session to begin with	
Stage	**Where to start**
You have done no resistance based strength training on a regular basis	If so, that makes you a novice – start with the stability sessions before progressing to strength then power
You have been doing resistance based strength training for 6–12 months and can do a perfect overhead squat	If so, that makes you experienced – you might benefit from doing the stability sessions, but you can start with the strength sessions before progressing to the power sessions
You have been doing resistance based strength training including some with kettlebells for 12 months or more and can do a perfect overhead squat	If so, you might benefit from doing the stability and strength sessions, but you can start with the power sessions.

the warm-up

Before you start any of the workouts, you need to do a warm-up. This can vary depending upon where you are – in a gym you might choose to use the cardio equipment (treadmill, rower, cross trainer) to get ready. This is fine, however I find the most effective warm-up is one that specifically mimics the work that is just about to be done, so I like to prepare by going through movements that feature in the actual workout. So at the start of the portfolio of moves I have included six exercises which are both simple and a productive means of preparing you for the types of movements and dynamic forces your body will experience during the workouts. Perform all the dynamic warm-up moves for between 30 and 60 seconds prior to working out with kettlebells.

post-workout stretch

In the world of fitness we habitually stretch at the end of our workout sessions when the muscles are still warm. However, muscles will also be fatigued and therefore not particularly receptive to being stretched. The reality is that most people just want to get out of the door when they have finished the workout section, and they view stretching as something that delays their shower, so I like to do the essential stretches just after the workout then make time when less fatigued to do some more quality, focused flexibility work.

The effects of stretching are cumulative so don't expect miracles the first time, or if you really struggle to make time for them, remember that the reason for warming up and stretching at the end of every session is to reduce the risk of injury. So, make a habit of incorporating stretching into your workout, or risk paying for the privilege of a physiotherapist telling you the same thing in the future.

You should complete the following essential stretches at the end of every kettlebell session (see below). Hold each of the stretches for at least 20 seconds and try to relax and enjoy them.

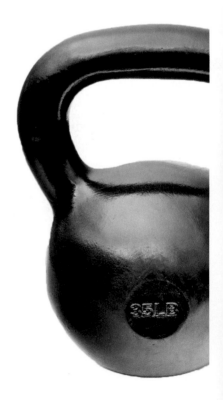

stretch 1 modified hurdle stretch

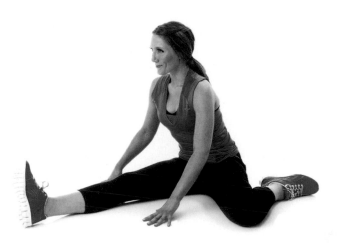

stretch 2 hip stretch

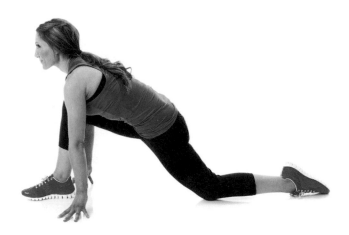

stretch 3 inner thigh

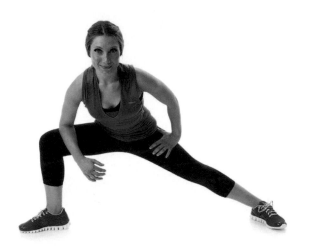

stretch 4 back extension

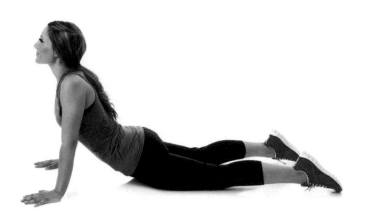

stretch 5 down dog

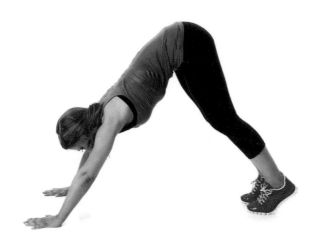

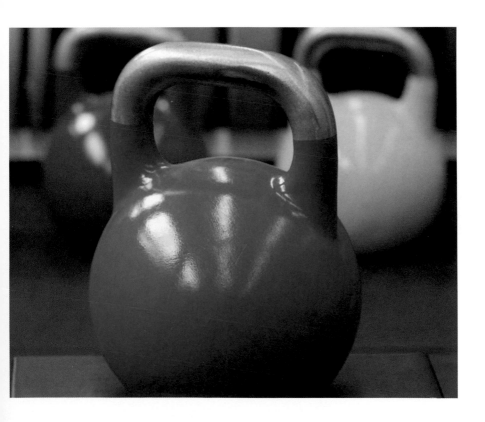

the workouts

the dynamic warm-up

The dynamic warm-up precedes all of the kettlebell workout sessions. Perform each of the warm-up moves in sequence for at least 30–60 seconds per move.

- Roll up roll down
- Deep squat
- Hip hinge
- Heel reaches
- Dynamic shoulder swings
- Hip thrusters

stability workout sessions

All of the stability moves are performed at a natural speed with the concentric and eccentric phase (muscle contract and release phase) taking the same amount of time.

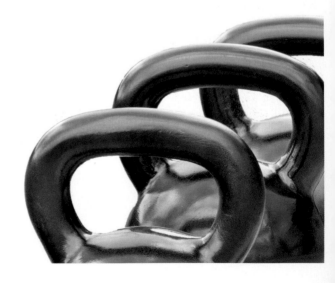

15 minute stability (30–60 seconds per move ● 1 set ● 2 circuits)

Order in which to do moves	Technique
exercise 7 one arm row (page 57)	
exercise 8 front squat (page 58)	
exercise 9 upright row (page 59)	
exercise 12 hip hinge with kettlebell (page 62)	
exercise 14 one handed floor press (page 64)	
exercise 17 single arm swing (page 67)	

20 minute stability (30–60 seconds per move ● 1 set ● 2 circuits)

Order in which to do moves	Technique
exercise 9 upright row (page 59)	
exercise 15 single leg side squat, kettlebell at chest (page 65)	
exercise 18 two arm swing (page 68)	
exercise 16 side bends; arms above head (page 66)	
exercise 10 outside foot pick-up (page 60)	
exercise 13 windmill dead lift (page 63)	

exercise 11 straight leg dead lift (page 61)	
exercise 17 single arm swing (page 67)	

30 minute stability (30–60 seconds per move ● 1 set ● 2 circuits)	
Order in which to do moves	**Technique**
exercise 13 windmill dead lift (page 63)	
exercise 14 one handed floor press (page 64)	
exercise 15 single leg side squat, kettlebell at chest (page 65)	

exercise 17 single arm swing (page 67)	
exercise 7 one arm row (page 57)	
exercise 10 outside foot pick-up (page 60)	
exercise 12 hip hinge with kettlebell (page 62)	
exercise 18 two arm swing (page 68)	
exercise 16 side bends, arms above head (page 66)	

exercise 8 front squat (page 58)	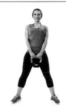

strength workout sessions

All of the Strength moves are performed at a natural speed with the concentric and eccentric phase (muscle contract and release phase) taking the same amount of time.

15 minute strength (30 seconds per move ● 1 set ● 2 circuits)	
Order in which to do moves	**Technique**
exercise 19 swing around the body (page 69)	
exercise 29 heel reach with kettlebell (page 79)	
exercise 20 shoulder press (page 70)	

exercise 21 overhead squat (page 71)	
exercise 22 swing clean, kettlebell to shoulder (page 72)	
exercise 32 push press with half squat (page 82)	
exercise 17 single arm swing (page 67)	

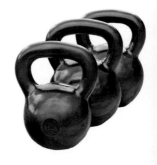

20 minute strength (45 seconds per move ● 1 set ● 3 circuits)	
Order in which to do moves	**Technique**
exercise 23 military press (page 73)	
exercise 25 single arm windmill (page 75)	
exercise 28 single leg dead lift, kettlebell to foot (page 78)	
exercise 30 pendulum swing 6–3 & 6–9 (page 80)	
exercise 31 single leg squat, kettlebell bottom up (page 81)	
exercise 34 halo circling kettlebell around head (page 85)	

exercise 35 sots press (page 86)	
exercise 17 single arm swing (page 67)	

30 minute strength (45 seconds per move ● 1 set ● 3 circuits)	
Order in which to do moves	**Technique**
exercise 17 single arm swing (page 67)	
exercise 27 clean and press (page 77)	
exercise 35 sots press (page 86)	

exercise 33 single leg hip hinge, kettlebell to foot (page 83)	
exercise 22 swing clean, kettlebell to shoulder (page 72)	
exercise 36 frontal swing, kettlebell between split stance legs (page 87)	
exercise 21 overhead squat (page 71)	
exercise 26 hammer curl (bicep curl, bottom up) (page 76)	
exercise 18 two arm swing (page 68)	

exercise 29 heel reach with kettlebell (page 79)	
exercise 32 push press with half squat (page 82)	

power workout sessions

All of the Power moves are performed at an increased speed compared to the Stability and Strength moves, with the concentric phase being performed faster than the eccentric phase.

15 minute power (20 seconds per move ● 2 sets ● 2 circuits)	
Order in which to do moves	**Technique**
exercise 37 dead lift clean (page 89)	
exercise 17 single arm swing (page 67)	

exercise 48 squat snatch (page 102)	
exercise 52 pendulum swing non-stop (page 107)	
exercise 39 plunges holding by the horns (page 91)	
exercise 43 coronal arc (hammer twist) (page 96)	
exercise 47 one handed swing, release and catch (page 101)	

20 minute power (20 seconds per move ● 2 sets ● 3 circuits)	
Order in which to do moves	**Technique**
exercise 40 one handed cross chop (page 92)	
exercise 17 single arm swing (page 67)	
exercise 44 the jerk (page 97)	
exercise 38 swing snatch, kettlebell above head (page 90)	
exercise 42 clean and step back (page 95)	
exercise 49 one arm swing and switch hands (page 103)	

exercise 50 bottom up snatch (page 104)	
exercise 45 skater swing (page 98)	
exercise 51 split jerk (page 106)	

30 minute power (30 seconds per move ● 3 sets ● 3 circuits)	
Order in which to do moves	**Technique**
exercise 38 swing snatch, kettlebell above head (page 90)	
exercise 17 single arm swing (page 67)	

exercise 41 the Andrea (page 93)	
exercise 51 split jerk (page 106)	
exercise 46 cross chop catch, step forward (page 100)	
exercise 45 skater swing (page 99)	
exercise 18 two arm swing (page 68)	
exercise 43 coronal arc (hammer twist) (page 96)	

exercise 48 squat snatch (page 102)	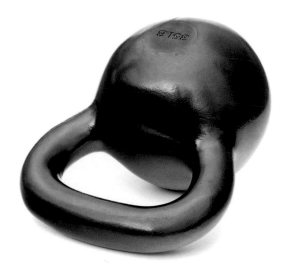
exercise 35 sots press (page 86)	

and finally...

The fantastic fitness industry that I work in has a habit of being able to reinvent the wheel at regular intervals. Kettlebells didn't need to be reinvented, but they did need to be tidied up and modernised so that they could be an appropriate training method for everybody rather than just the preserve of 'garage' gyms and strength competitors. They have managed to achieve this transformation in a very short time, going from being something that few people had ever used to being a key item of fitness equipment at home and in gymnasiums. The possibilities are endless and, no matter what your goals, used sensibly kettlebells can play a significant part in helping you to achieve them.

Whether you are a personal trainer, sportsperson or fitness enthusiast, I hope you are now far better informed about how to get the most out of the valuable time you spend doing exercise with your kettlebells, a most versatile and dynamic piece of equipment. All I ask is that you use all the information I have given in this book and make it part of an integrated health and fitness-driven lifestyle. My many thousands of hours spent in gymnasiums, health clubs, sport fields and with personal training clients has taught me that, given the chance, people like to do the things they are already good at. So before you reach your maximum potential, the smart ones among you will be looking to introduce new challenges with different equipment like dumbbells, barbells, medicine balls, gym balls and suspension system training, as well as new challenges for cardiovascular fitness and flexibility.

As a personal trainer I know that I have a greater than average interest in the human body and the effects of exercise, partly because it is my passion and partly because it is my job. I also recognise that in the busy world we live in, expecting the same level of interest and dedication from clients towards health and exercise is unrealistic, so for me the best personal trainers are those who help clients to integrate exercise into everyday life rather than allow it to dominate.

The body is an amazing thing and responds to exercise by adapting and improving the way that it functions. Exercise is not all about pain, challenges and hard work – hopefully, despite this being the overpowering reputation that kettlebells have, I have been able to help show you that this doesn't have to be the case– rather it is about making sure that in the long term your life includes the elements that have the greatest effect. I strongly believe that every minute you invest in exercise pays you back with interest, and that it's all about finding the right balance.

Finding that balance is different for all of us, but I think you can't go far wrong if you train for stability, strength and maybe power. Walk and run, eat healthily and drink water. Find time to relax and stretch, but above all remember: if you ever find yourself lacking in motivation, the best advice I can give anybody wanting to feel healthier is that if you're moving, you're improving.

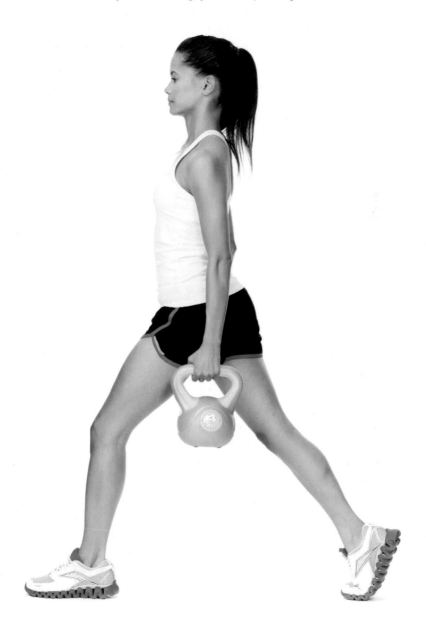

fitness glossary

As a person interested in health and fitness there is no need to sound like you have swallowed a textbook for breakfast. Yes, you need to understand how things work, but I feel there is more skill in being able to explain complicated subjects in simple language rather than simply memorising a textbook. The following glossary sets out to explain the key words and phrases that, for a person interested in the body, are useful to know and that will help you get the most out of this book, especially the training section.

Abdominals The name given to the group of muscles that make up the front of the torso, also known as 'the abs'.

Abduction The opposite of adduction (see below). The term the medical profession uses to describe any movement of a limb away from the midline of the body. So, if you raise your arm up to the side, that would be described as 'abduction of the shoulder'.

Acceleration The opposite of deceleration (see below). The speed at which a movement increases from start to finish. When using weights, accelerating the weight when moving it at a constant speed really adds to the challenge.

Adduction The opposite of abduction (see above). The term the medical profession uses to describe any movement of a limb across the midline of the body. So, if you cross your legs that would be 'adduction of the hip'.

Aerobic The opposite of anaerobic (see below). The word invented in 1968 by Dr Kenneth Cooper to describe the process in our body when we are working 'with oxygen'. While the term is now associated with the dance-based exercise to music (ETM), the original aerobic exercises that Cooper measured were cross country running, skiing, swimming, running, cycling and walking. Generally most people consider activity up to 80 per cent of maximum heart rate (MHR, see below) to be aerobic and beyond that to be anaerobic.

Age The effects of exercise change throughout life. With strength training in particular age will influence the outcome. As you reach approximately the age of 40, maintaining and developing lean muscle mass becomes harder and, in fact, the body starts to lose lean mass as a natural part of the ageing process. This can be combated somewhat with close attention to diet and exercise. At the other end of the scale a sensible approach is required when introducing very young people to training with weights.

Personally I don't like to see children participating in very heavy weight training, as it should not be pursued by boys and girls who are still growing (in terms of bone structure, rather than muscle structure), as excessive loading on prepubescent bones may have an adverse effect. There is very little conclusive research available on this subject, as it would require children to be put through tests that require them to lift very heavy weights in order to assess how much is too much. Newborn babies have over 300 bones and as we grow some bones fuse together leaving an adult with an average of 206 mature bones by age 20.

Agility Your progressive ability to move at speed and change direction while doing so.

Anaerobic The opposite of aerobic (see above). High intensity bursts of cardio-vascular activity generally above 80 per cent of MHR. The term literally means 'without oxygen' because when operating at this speed, the body flicks over to the fuel stored in muscles rather than mixing the fuel first with oxygen, which is what happens during aerobic activity.

Anaerobic threshold The point at which the body cannot clear lactic acid fast enough to avoid a build-up in the bloodstream. The delaying of this occurrence is a major characteristic of performance athletes, their frequent high intensity training increases (delays) the point at which this waste product becomes overwhelming.

Assessment I like to say that if you don't assess, you guess, so before embarking on any exercise regime you should assess your health and fitness levels in a number of areas, which can include flexibility, range of motion, strength or any of the cardiac outputs that can be measured at home or in the laboratory.

Barbell A long bar (6–7ft) with disc weights loaded onto each end. Olympic bars are competition grade versions that rotate on bearings to enable very heavy weights to be lifted.

Biceps The muscle at the front of the arm. It makes up about one-third of the entire diameter of the upper arm with the triceps forming the other two-thirds.

Blood pressure When the heart contracts and squirts out blood the pressure on the walls of the blood vessels is the blood pressure. It is expressed as a fraction, for example 130/80. The 130 (systolic) is the high point of the pressure being exerted on the tubes and the 80 (diastolic) is the lower amount of pressure between the main pulses.

Body Pump® This is a group exercise programme available in health clubs that changed the way people think about lifting weights simply by using music for timing and motivation. Rather than counting the reps, the class follows the set tunes and work around all the different muscle groups as the music tracks change.

Cardiovascular system (CV) This is the superhighway around the body. Heart, lungs and blood vessels transport and deliver the essentials of life: oxygen, energy, nutrients. Having delivered all this good stuff it then removes the rubbish by transporting away the waste products from the complex structure of muscle tissue.

Centre line This is an imaginary line that runs down the centre of the body from the chin to a point through the ribs, pelvis, right down to the floor.

Circuit A list of exercises can be described as a circuit. If you see '2 circuits' stated on a programme, it means you are expected to work through that list of exercises twice.

Concentric contraction The opposite of eccentric contraction (see below). If this word isn't familiar to you just think 'contract', as in to get smaller/shorter.

A concentric contraction is when a muscle shortens under tension. For example, when you lift a cup towards your mouth you produce a concentric contraction of the bicep (don't make the mistake of thinking that when you lower the cup it's a concentric contraction of the opposite muscle, i.e. the triceps, as it isn't ... it's an eccentric movement of the bicep).

Contact points The parts of the body that are touching the bench, ball, wall or floor. The smaller the contact points, e.g. heels rather than entire foot, the greater the balance and stabilisation requirements of an exercise.

Core Ah, the core. Ask 10 trainers to describe the core and you will get 10 different answers. To me it is the obvious muscles of the abdominals, the lower back, etc., but it is also the smaller deep muscles and connective tissue that provide stability and strength to the individual. Muscles such as the glutes, hamstrings and, most importantly, the pelvic floor are often forgotten as playing a key role in the core. When I am doing a demonstration of core muscle activation, the way I sum up the core is that the majority of movements that require stability are in some way using all of the muscles that connect between the nipples and the knees.

Creatine An amino acid created naturally in your body. Every time you perform any intense exercise, e.g. weight training, your body uses creatine as a source of energy. The body has the ability to store more creatine than it produces, so taking it as a supplement would allow you to train for longer at high intensity. Consuming creatine is only productive when combined with high intensity training and, therefore, is not especially relevant until you start to train for power.

Cross training An excellent approach to fitness training where you use a variety of methods to improve your fitness rather than just one. Cross training is now used by athletes and sportspeople to reduce injury levels, as it ensures that you have a balanced amount of cardio, strength and flexibility in a schedule.

Deceleration The opposite of acceleration (see above). It is the decrease in velocity of an object. If you consider that injuries in sportspeople more often occur during the deceleration phase rather than the acceleration phase of their activity (for example, a sprinter pulling up at the end of the race rather than when they push out of the starting blocks), you will focus particularly on this phase of all the moves in this book. The power moves especially call for you to control the 'slowing down' part of the move, which requires as much skill as it does to generate the speed in the first place.

Delayed onset muscle soreness (DOMS) This is that unpleasant muscle soreness that you get after starting a new kind of activity or when you have worked harder than normal. It was once thought that the soreness was caused by lactic acid becoming 'trapped' in the muscle after a workout, but we now realise that this is simply not the case because lactic acid doesn't hang around – it is continuously moved and metabolised. The pain is far more likely to be caused by a mass of tiny little muscle tears. It's not a cure, but some light exercise will often ease the pain because this increases the flow of blood and nutrients to the damaged muscle tissue.

Deltoid A set of three muscles that sit on top of your shoulders.

Dumbbell A weight designed to be lifted with one hand. It can be adjustable or of a fixed weight, and the range of weight available goes a rather pointless 1kg up to a massive 50kg plus.

Dynamometer A little gadget used to measure strength by squeezing a handheld device that then measures the force of your grip.

Dyna-Band® A strip of rubber used as an alternative to a dumbbell, often by physiotherapists for working muscles through specific ranges of motion where weights are either too intense or can't target the appropriate muscles. Dyna-Band® can be held flat against the skin to give subtle muscle stimulation, for example, by wrapping a strip around the shoulders (like an Egyptian mummy), you can then work through protraction and retraction movements of the shoulder girdle.

Eccentric contraction The opposite of concentric contraction (see above). The technical term for when a muscle is lengthening under tension. An easy example to remember is the lowering of a dumbbell during a bicep curl, which is described as an eccentric contraction of the bicep.

Eye line Where you are looking when performing movements. Some movement patterns are significantly altered by correct or incorrect eye line, for example, if the eye line is too high during squats, then the head is lifted and the spine will experience excessive extension.

Fascia Connective tissue that attaches muscles to muscles and enables individual muscle fibres to be bundled together. While not particularly scientific, a good way to visualise fascia is that it performs in a similar way to the skin of a sausage by keeping its contents where it should be.

Fitball (gym ball, stability ball, Swiss ball) The large balls extensively used for stability training by therapists and in gyms. They are available in sizes 55–75cm. If you are using them for weight training always remember to add your weight and the dumbbell weight together to make sure the total weight doesn't exceed the safety limit of the ball.

Flexibility The misconception is that we do flexibility to actually stretch the muscle fibres and make them longer, whereas, in fact, when we stretch effectively it is the individual muscle fibres that end up moving more freely against each other, creating a freer increased range of motion.

Foam rolling This is a therapy technique that has become mainstream. You use a round length of foam to massage your own muscles (generally you sit or lie on the roller to exert force via your bodyweight). Interestingly, while this has a positive effect on your muscle fibres, it is the fascia that is 'stretched' most. Foam rolling is actually rather painful when you begin, but as you improve, the pain decreases. Often used by athletes as part of their warm-up.

Free weights The collective name for dumbbells and barbells. There has been a huge influx of new products entering this category so in the free weights area of a good gym you will also find kettlebells and medicine balls. In bodybuilding gyms you will often find items not designed for exercise but which are challenging to lift and use, such as heavy chains, ropes and tractor tyres.

Functional training Really all training should be functional as it is the pursuit of methods and movements that benefit you in day to day life. Therefore, doing squats are functionally beneficial for your abdominals because they work them in conjunction with other muscles, but sit-ups are not because they don't work the abdominals in a way that relates to many everyday movements.

Gait Usually associated with running and used to describe the way that a runner hits the ground either with the inside, centre or outside of their foot and, specifically, how the foot, ankle and knee joints move. However, this term always relates to how you stand and walk. Mechanical issues that exist below the knee can have a knock-on effect on other joints and muscles throughout the body. Pronation is the name given to the natural inward roll of the ankle that occurs when the heel strikes the ground and the foot flattens out. Supination refers to the opposite outward roll that occurs during the push-off phase of the walking and running movement. A mild amount of pronation and supination is both healthy and necessary to propel the body forward.

Genes As in the hereditary blueprint that you inherited from your parents, rather than the blue denim variety. Genes can influence everything from your hair colour to your predisposition to developing diseases. Clearly there is nothing you can do to influence your genes, so accept that some athletes are born great because they have the odds stacked on their side while others have to train their way to glory.

Gluteus maximus A set of muscles on your bottom, also known as 'the glutes'.

Hamstring A big set of muscles down the back of the thigh. It plays a key role in core stability and needs to be flexible if you are to develop a good squat technique.

Heart rate (HR) Also called 'the pulse'. It is the number of times each minute that your heart contracts. An athlete's HR could be as low as 35 beats per minute (BPM) when resting but can also go up to 250BPM during activity.

Hypertrophy The growth of skeletal muscle. This is what a bodybuilder is constantly trying to do. The number of muscle fibres we have is fixed, so rather than 'growing' new muscles fibres hypertrophy is the process of increasing the size of the existing fibre. Building muscle is a slow and complex process that requires constant training and a detailed approach to nutrition.

Insertion All muscles are attached to bone or other muscles by tendons or fascia. The end of the muscle that moves during a contraction is the insertion, with the moving end being called the origin. Note that some muscles have more than one origin and insertion.

Integration (compound) The opposite of isolation (see below). Movement that requires more than one joint and muscle to be involved, e.g. a squat.

Isolation The opposite of integration (see above). A movement that requires only one joint and muscle to be involved, e.g. a bicep curl.

Interval training A type of training where you do blocks of high intensity exercise followed by a block of lower intensity (recovery) exercise. The blocks can be time based or marked by distance (in cardio training). Interval training is highly beneficial to both athletes and fitness enthusiasts as it allows them to subject their body to high intensity activity in short achievable bursts.

Intra-abdominal pressure (IAP) An internal force that assists in the stabilization of the lumber spine. This relates to the collective effects of pressure exerted on the structures of the diaphragm, transversus abdominis, multifidi and the pelvic floor.

Kettlebells In its original form a kettlebell was a cannonball with a handle on it. Modern versions are either know as 'classic' or 'pro grade' competition kettlebells. The weight of kettlebells has traditionally been measured in 'poods' (a word derived from the Russian for 'Russian pound'), which equates to roughly 16kg to

1 pood. For beginners this is a challenging weight so, as kettlebells have become increasingly 'mass market', manufacturers have introduced lighter versions.

Most gyms will be equipped with cast iron or steel kettlebells ranging from 8kg to 332kg. If the kettlebells all vary in size, they are 'classic' kettlebells, but if they are all the same size irrespective of what weight they are, then they are probably what is classed as being 'competition' or 'pro grade'. This means that no matter what weight you are lifting the dimensions of the weights are all the same. This is important to people who enter lifting competitions because they can develop their technique using the standard shape and not have to re-learn or change their methods as they progress to heavier weights. The 'pro grade' kettlebells also have slimmer smoother handles which help to minimise fatigue in your grip when performing high repetition sets.

Kinesiology The scientific study of the movement of our anatomical structure. It was only in the 1960s with the creation of fixed weight machines that we started to isolate individual muscles and work them one at a time. This is a step backwards in terms of kinesiology because in real life a single muscle rarely works in isolation.

Kinetic chain The series of reactions/forces throughout the nerves, bones, muscles, ligaments and tendons when the body moves or has a force applied against it.

Kyphosis Excessive curvature of the human spine. This can range from being a little bit round shouldered to being in need of corrective surgery.

Lactic acid A by-product of muscle contractions. If lactic acid reaches a level higher than that which the body can quickly clear from the blood stream, the person has reached their anaerobic threshold. Training at high intensity has the effect of delaying the point at which lactic acid levels cause fatigue.

Latissimus dorsi Two triangular-shaped muscles that run from the top of the neck and spine to the back of the upper arm and all the way into the lower back, also known as 'the lats'.

Ligaments Connective tissues that attach bone to bone or cartilage to bone. They have fewer blood vessels passing through them than muscles, which makes them whiter (they look like gristle) and also slower to heal.

Lordosis Excessive curvature of the lower spine. Mild cases that are diagnosed early can often be resolved through core training and by working on flexibility with exercises best prescribed by a physiotherapist.

Massage Not just for pleasure or relaxation, this can speed up recovery and reduce discomfort after a hard training session. Massage can help maintain range of motion in joints and reduce mild swelling caused by injury related inflammation.

Magnesium An essential mineral that plays a role in over 300 processes in the body including in the cardiovascular system and tissue repair.

Maximum heart rate (MHR) The highest number of times the heart can contract (or beat) in one minute. A very approximate figure can be obtained for adults by using the following formula: 220 – current age = MHR. Athletes often exceed this guideline, but only because they have progressively pushed themselves and increased their strength over time.

Medicine ball Traditionally this was a leather ball packed with fibre to make it heavy. Modern versions are solid rubber or filled with a heavy gel.

Mobility The ability of a joint to move freely through a range of motion. Mobility is very important because if you have restricted joint mobility and with exercise you start to load that area with weights, the chances are that you will compound the problem.

Muscular endurance (MSE) The combination of strength and endurance. The ability to perform many repetitions against a given resistance for a prolonged period. In strength training any more than 12 reps is considered MSE.

Negative-resistance training (NRT) Resistance training in which the muscles lengthen while still under tension. Lowering a barbell, bending down and running downhill are all examples. It is felt that this type of training will increase muscle size more quickly than other types of training, but if you only ever do NRT you won't be training the body to develop usable functional strength.

Obliques The muscles on both sides of the abdomen that rotate and flex the torso. Working these will have no effect on 'love handles', which are fat that sits above, but is not connected to, the obliques.

Origin All muscles are attached to bone or others muscles by tendons or fascia. The end of the muscle which is not moved during a contraction is the origin, with the moving end being called the insertion. Note that some muscles have more than one origin and insertion.

Overtraining Excessive amounts of exercise, intensity, or both volume and intensity of training, resulting in fatigue, illness, injury and/or impaired performance. Overtraining can occur in individual parts of the body or throughout, which is a good reason for keeping records of the training you do so you can see if patterns of injuries relate to a certain time or types of training you do throughout the year.

Patience With strength training – more than any other type of exercise – patience is essential. When you exercise the results are based on the ability of the body to 'change', which includes changes in the nervous system as well as progressive improvements in the soft tissues (muscles, ligaments and tendons). While it is not instantly obvious why patience is so important, it becomes clearer when you consider how, for example, the speed of change differs in the blood rich muscles at a faster rate than the more avascular ligaments and tendons. Improvements take time so be patient.

Pectorals The muscles of the chest, also known as 'the pecs'. Working the pecs will have a positive effect on the appearance of the chest, however, despite claims, it is unlikely that working the pecs will have any effect on the size of female breasts although it can make them feel firmer if the muscle tone beneath them is increased.

Pelvic floor (PF) Five layers of muscle and connective tissue at the base of the torso. The male and female anatomy differs in this area, however strength and endurance is essential in the PF for both men and women if you are to attain maximum strength in the core. Most of the core training or stability products work the PF.

Periodisation Sums up the difference between a long-term strategy and short-term gains. Periodisation is where you plan to train the body for different outcomes throughout a year or longer. The simplest version of this method would be where a track athlete worked on muscle strength and growth during the winter and then speed and maintenance of muscle endurance during the summer racing session.

Planes of motion The body moves through three planes of motion. Sagittal describes all the forward and back movement; frontal describes the side to side movements; and transverse describes the rotational movements. In everyday life most of the movements we go through involve actions from all three planes all of the time – it is really only 'artificial' techniques, such as bicep curls and deltoid raises, that call upon just one plane at a time.

Plyometrics An explosive movement practised by athletes, for example, two footed jumps over hurdles. This is not for beginners or those with poor levels of flexibility and/or a limited range of motion.

Prone Lying face down, also the standard description of exercises performed from a lying face down position. The opposite of supine (see below).

Protein A vital nutrient that needs to be consumed every day. Carbohydrates provide your body with energy, while protein helps your muscles to recover and repair more quickly after exercise. Foods high in protein include whey protein, which is a by-product of the dairy industry and is consumed as a shake, fish, chicken, eggs, dairy produce (such as milk, cheese and yoghurt), beef and soya.

Increased activity will increase your protein requirements. A lack of quality protein can result in loss of muscle tissue and tone, a weaker immune system, slower recovery and lack of energy. The protein supplements industry has developed many convenient methods for consuming protein in the form of powders, shakes and food bars, most of which contain the most easily digested and absorbable type of protein, whey protein.

Pyramid A programming method for experienced weight trainers. A set of the same exercises are performed at least three times, each set has progressively fewer repetitions in it, but greater resistance. When you reach the peak of the pyramid (heaviest weight) you then perform the same three sets again in reverse order. For example, going up the pyramid would ask for 15 reps with 10kg, 10 reps with 15kg, 5 reps with 20kg. Going down the pyramid would require 10 reps with 15kg, 15 reps with 10kg.

Quadriceps The groups of muscles at the front of the thighs, also known as 'the quads'. They are usually the first four muscle names that personal trainers learn, but just in case you have forgotten the four are: vastus intermedius, rectus femoris (that's the one that's also a hip flexor), vastus lateralis and vastus medialis.

Range of motion (ROM) The degree of movement that occurs at one of the body's joints. Without physio equipment it is difficult to measure a joint precisely, however you can easily compare the shoulder, spine, hip, knee and ankle on the left side with the range of motion of the same joints on the right side.

Reebok Core Board® A stability product that you predominately stand on. The platform has a central axis which creates a similar experience to using a wobble board, however, the Reebok Core Board® also rotates under tension so you can train against torsion and recoil.

Recoil The elastic characteristic of muscle when 'stretched' to return the body parts back to the start positions after a dynamic movement.

Recovery/rest The period when not exercising and the most important component of any exercise programme. It is only during rest periods that the body adapts to previous training loads and rebuilds itself to be stronger, thereby facilitating improvement. Rest is therefore vitally important for progression.

Repetitions How many of each movement you do, also known as 'reps'. On training programmes you will have seen three numerical figures that you need to understand – reps, sets and circuits.

Repetition max (RM) The maximum load that a muscle or muscle group can lift. Establishing your 1RM can help you select the right amount of weight for different exercises and it is also a good way of monitoring progress.

Resistance training Any type of training with weights, including gym machines, barbells and dumbbells and bodyweight exercises.

Resting heart rate (RHR) The number of contractions (heartbeats) per minute when at rest. The average RHR for an adult is approx 72BPM, but for athletes it can be much lower.

Scapula retraction Not literally 'pulling your shoulders back', but that is a good cue to use to get this desired effect. Many people develop rounded shoulders, which when lifting weights puts them at a disadvantage because the scapular cannot move freely, so by lifting the ribs and squeezing the shoulder blades back the shoulder girdle is placed in a good lifting start position.

Sciatica Layman's term for back pain which radiates through the spine, buttocks and hamstrings. Usually due to pressure on the sciatic nerve being shortened, which runs from the lower back and down the legs, rather than being a problem with the skeleton. Most often present in people who sit a lot. Core training, massage and flexibility exercises can frequently cure the problem.

Set A block of exercises usually put together to work an area of the body to the point of fatigue, so if you were working legs you may do squats, lunges and calf raises straight after each other, then repeat them again for a second 'set'.

Speed, agility and quickness (SAQ)® Although in fact a brand name, this has become the term used to describe a style of exercises or drills which are designed to improve speed, agility and quickness. Very athletic and dynamic, often including plyometric movements.

Stability ball (also gym ball, fitball and Swiss ball) The large balls extensively used for suitability training by therapists and in gyms. They are available in sizes 55–75cm. If you are using them for weight training always remember to add your weight and the dumbbell (or kettlebell) weight together to make sure the total weight doesn't exceed the safety limit of the ball.

Stretch A balanced approach to stretching is one of the most important elements of feeling good and reducing the likelihood of developing non-trauma soft tissue injuries. When we lift weight clearly the muscle fatigues and as a result at the end of the session the overall muscle (rather than individual fibres) can feel 'tight' or shortened. Doing a stretch will help return the muscle to itspre-exercise state. Dynamic stretching (rhythmic movements to promote optimum range of movement from muscle/joints) should be performed pre-workout. Static stretching performed after the kettlebell session is productive as long as you dedicate enough time to each position, so give each section of the body worked at least 90 seconds of attention.

Suspension training A strength training format that allows you to use your bodyweight as the resistance by means of hanging from long adjustable straps that are suspended above head height, also known as 'TRX®'. By adjusting the length of the straps and changing the body and foot position the challenge can be adapted for all levels of ability.

Superset Similar to a set, but each sequential exercise is performed with no rest in between. The moves in a superset are selected to ensure that they relate to each other, for example, an exercise that focused on shoulders and triceps, such as a shoulder press, would be followed by another shoulder/triceps move, such as dips.

Supine Lying face up, also the standard description of exercises performed from a lying face up position. The opposite of prone (see above).

Tendon Connective tissue that attaches muscles to bones. Muscle and tendon tissue merge together progressively, rather than there being a clear line where tendon starts and muscle finishes. Like ligaments, a tendon has fewer blood vessels running through it and is less flexible than muscle tissue.

Time As a personal trainer, I have been asked many times, 'What is the best time of day to exercise?' The answer depends. If you are an athlete training almost every day perhaps twice a day, then I would say that strength training in the morning could be more productive than at other times due to the body clock and fluctuating hormone levels throughout the day. However, if the question is asked by a casual exerciser with an average diet and a job and busy lifestyle, my answer would be to exercise at any time of the day, as exercise is a productive use of your valuable free time.

Torsion Stress on the body when external forces twist it about the spinal axis.

Training partner A training partner can be a person who keeps you company and motivates you while you exercise or they can also take the role of being your 'spotter' when you are lifting heavy weights. The role of a spotter is to hand and take the weights from you when you are fatigued from a heavy set of lifts. Choose your partner wisely; weights can be dangerous, so ensure they take the responsibility seriously.

Training shoes The best shoes to wear when lifting weights will have a combination of good grip and stability. Some athletes are now choosing to lift while wearing no or very thin soled shoes on the basis that it will work the muscles in their feet more and therefore give greater results – if you do consider doing this, take a number of weeks to build up the amount you do barefoot to give the feet time to strengthen slowly. Athletes competing in powerlifting contests will

. . . .

wear performance shoes that give their feet increased support, however, these are not suitable for exercises in which the foot is moved.

Transversus abdominis A relatively thin sheet of muscle which wraps around the torso. This is the muscle that many people think they activate by following the instruction of 'pull your stomach in', however, that movement is more likely to be facilitated by the main abdominals. For your information, a flat stomach is more likely to be achieved by simply standing up straight, as this ensures the correct distance between the ribs and pelvis.

Triceps Muscles at the back of the upper arms. They make up approximately two-thirds of the diameter of the upper arm, so if arm size is your goal, working the triceps will be a priority.

Vertebrae Individual bones that make up the spinal column. The intervertebral discs that sit between them are there to keep the vertebrae separated, cushion the spine and protect the spinal cord.

VO$_2$ max The highest volume of oxygen a person can infuse into their blood during exercise. A variety of calculations or tests can be used to establish your VO$_2$ max; these include measuring the heart rate during and post aerobic activity. As each of these tests includes a measurement of the distance covered as well as the heart's reaction to activity, the most popular methods of testing VO$_2$ max are running, stepping, swimming or cycling for a set time and distance.

Warm-up The first part of any workout session that is intended to prepare the body for the exercise ahead of it. I find it is best to take the lead from the sports world and base the warm-up exactly on the movements you will do in the session. So if you are about to do weights rather than jog, go through some of the movements unloaded to prepare the body for the ranges of motion you will later be doing loaded.

Warm-down The slowing down or controlled recovery period after a workout session. A warm-down can include low level cardio work to return the heart rate to a normal speed as well as stretching and relaxation.

Wobble board A circular wooden disc that you stand on with a hemisphere on one side. Originally used just by physiotherapists, they are now common in gyms and are used for stability training, core exercises and strengthening the ankle and/or rehabilitation from ankle injuries. Technology has been applied to this simple piece of equipment and you now have progressive devices such as the Reebok Core Board® and the BOSU® (Both Sides Up), which achieve the same and more than the wooden versions.

X-training, activity. See cross training (above).

Yoga Probably the oldest form of fitness training in existence. Yoga has many different types (or styles) ranging from very passive stretching techniques through to explosive and dynamic style. It is often associated with hippy culture and 'yummy mummies', however, if you are doing any type of strength training, yoga will compliment this nicely.

about the author

STEVE BARRETT is a former national competitor in athletics, rugby, mountain biking and sport aerobics. His career in the fitness industry as a personal trainer spans over 20 years. His work as a lecturer and presenter has taken him to 34 countries including the United States, Russia and Australia.

For many years Steve delivered Reebok International's fitness strategy and implementation via their training faculty Reebok University. He gained the title of Reebok Global Master Trainer, which is a certification that required a minimum of three years' studying, presenting and researching both practical and academic subjects. Between the years 2000 and 2008 in this role he lectured and presented to more than 20,000 fellow fitness professionals and students.

Steve played a key role in the development of the training systems and launch of two significant products in the fitness industry: the Reebok Deck and Reebok Core Board®. As a personal trainer, in addition to teaching the teachers and working with the rich and famous he has been involved in the training of many international athletes and sports personalities at Liverpool FC, Arsenal FC, Manchester United FC, the Welsh RFU, and UK athletics.

Within the fitness industry he has acted as a consultant to leading brand names, including Nestlé, Kelloggs, Reebok and Adidas.

His media experience includes being guest expert for the BBC and writing for numerous publications including *The Times*, *The Independent*, *The Daily Telegraph*, *Runner's World*, *Men's Fitness*, *Rugby News*, *Health & Fitness*, *Zest*, *Ultra-FIT*, *Men's Health UK* and *Australia* and many more.

Steve's expertise is in the development of logical, user friendly, safe and effective training programmes. The work that he is most proud of, however, isn't his celebrity projects, but the changes to ordinary people's lives that never get reported.

Now that he has been teaching fitness throughout his 20s, 30s and now 40s, he has developed a tremendous ability to relate to the challenges that people face to incorporate exercise into their lifestyle, and while the fitness industry expects personal trainers to work with clients for a short period of time, Steve has been working with many of his clients for nearly two decades, continuously evolving to meet their changing needs. His fun and direct approach has resulted in many couch potatoes running out of excuses and transforming into fitness converts.

www.Trade-Secrets-of-a-Personal-Trainer.com

index